REVERSING
ATHEROSCLEROSIS

Publication Number 1031

AMERICAN LECTURE SERIES®

A Monograph in

AMERICAN LECTURES IN LIVING CHEMISTRY

Edited by

I. NEWTON KUGELMASS, M.D., Ph.D., Sc.D.

*Consultant to the Departments of Health and Hospitals
New York, New York*

REVERSING
ATHEROSCLEROSIS

By

G. A. GRESHAM, T.D., M.D., Sc.D., F.R.C. Path.

Professor of Morbid Anatomy and Histopathology
University of Cambridge
Fellow of Jesus College
Cambridge, England

82 9596

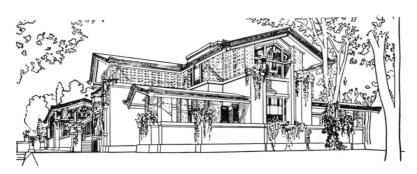

CHARLES C THOMAS • PUBLISHER
Springfield • Illinois • U.S.A.

Published and Distributed Throughout the World by
CHARLES C THOMAS ● PUBLISHER
Bannerstone House
301-327 East Lawrence Avenue, Springfield, Illinois, U.S.A.

© *1980, by* CHARLES C THOMAS ● PUBLISHER
ISBN 0-398-03931-3
Library of Congress Catalog Card Number: 79-12622

With THOMAS BOOKS *careful attention is given to all details of manufacturing and design. It is the Publisher's desire to present books that are satisfactory as to their physical qualities and artistic possibilities and appropriate for their particular use.* THOMAS BOOKS *will be true to those laws of quality that assure a good name and good will.*

Printed in the United States of America
V-R-1

Library of Congress Cataloging in Publication Data
Gresham, Geoffrey Austin.
 Reversing atherosclerosis.

 (American lecture series ; no. 1031)
 Includes index.
 1. Atherosclerosis. 2. Atherosclerosis--Prevention.
I. Title. [DNLM: 1. Arteriosclerosis. WG550 G831r]
RC692.G73   616.1'36   79-12622
ISBN 0-398-03931-3

PREFACE

MORTALITY data in the United Kingdom have shown a decline in the total death rate of persons aged thirty to seventy-five.[1] This change has been accompanied by an alteration in the pattern of the causes of death in that the proportion of deaths assigned to ischaemic heart disease has risen sharply. Among men aged forty-five to forty-nine, 40 percent of deaths were due to heart disease in 1971, whereas 20 percent were so ascribed in 1951. This phenomenon might be partly due to revisions of the International Classification of Diseases. Even when this point was taken into account, it became clear that the mortality had risen steeply among men and in particular among young men where the mortality from ischaemic heart disease was 80 percent higher in 1973 than in 1950.

Figures such as these and the fact that ischaemic heart disease is now the most common cause of death in adult Western males suggest that variable factors operate in the production of coronary artery disease. The problem is to define the point at which they operate. A mortality statistic such as ischaemic heart disease means that death was due to impaired myocardial nutrition. It could be that the myocardium of modern males has become more susceptible to ischaemia or that the incidence of occlusive coronary atherosclerosis is increasing in younger men. Another explanation could be that the incidence of coronary artery thrombosis is increased.

Whatever the explanation, the factors that promote ischaemic heart disease should be defined and, if possible, their mode of action investigated. Much of this work has been done in this century both in man and in the experimental animal. The Proceedings of the Third International Symposium on Athero-

---

[1]Death from ischaemic heart disease. *Br Med J*, ii:537, 1977.

v

sclerosis bring together much that had been done up to 1974.[2] This comprehensive record, however, contains little to do with the possibility that atherosclerosis might regress; this is not surprising since studies on this matter have only come about in relatively recent times. Such work is a logical development of the extensive studies of induction of atherosclerosis that have been made over the years.

There are some who deny that there is any evidence of regression of atherosclerosis in man and that animal studies demonstrating regression are irrelevant to the human situation.[3] The purpose of this book is to challenge this view by an examination of retrospective evidence in man, followed by an account of the occluding arterial lesion and, most importantly, its mode of origin. Each component of the lesion will be examined to define the processes that cause it to accumulate and the potential factors that might lead to reversal of the lesion. Tissue culture work on the cells of the arterial wall also provides indications of atherogenic mechanisms and avenues that might be explored to implement regression.

A good deal of work has already been done in experimental animals to study the effects of withdrawal of known risk factors. This and reports of attempts at drug therapy will occupy a later part of the book.

Much of the criticism about regressive studies has been levelled at the methods used to quantitate lesions both *in vivo* and at postmortem examination. A chapter is devoted to the methods and to modern developments that enable an accurate assessment of occlusive arterial disease in man.

[2]Schettler, F. G. and Weizel, A.: Atherosclerosis III. Proceedings of the Third International Symposium. Berlin, Springer-Verlag, 1974.
[3]Progression and regression of atherosclerosis. *Br Med J*, i:481, 1976.

CONTENTS

vii

REVERSING
ATHEROSCLEROSIS

CHAPTER 1

RETROSPECTIVE STUDIES ON REGRESSION OF HUMAN ATHEROSCLEROSIS

$\mathbf{R}$ECENT advances in molecular biology involving work on the active metabolism of various biological substances have led to radical changes in attitude by pathologists about the fate of tissue components. In 1924, Aschoff (1) proposed the idea that atherosclerosis might be reversible. At that time it seemed ludicrous to suggest that a degenerative process composed of layers of lipid, bits of collagen and calcium, and other things might be capable of resolution. Now the concept is acceptable.

Aschoff had noted a decline in the incidence of atherosclerotic disease in Central Europe after World War I and proposed the view that this was due to a reduced intake of dietary fat during the war years. In 1958, Katz et al. (2) reviewed a number of older reports that appeared to indicate that human atherosclerosis might be a reversible disorder. The problem with such reports was the lack of a clear definition of the disease being considered. Basically, the reports described decreases in cardiac infarction or in sudden cardiac death following severe dietary restrictions. It is not clear whether the effect was on coronary atherosclerosis, coronary thrombosis, or on myocardial susceptibility to dysrhythmic action. Furthermore, the dietary restriction that had taken place involved not only fat but other food constituents as well. There was a reduced intake of calories, protein, and other ingredients. Such deficiencies of one sort or another have been implicated in atherogenesis. Clearly, the interpretation of the precise mode of action of such polymorphic dietary restriction cannot be made easily.

Unfortunately, much of the epidemiological work in man has been retrospective and suffers from the defects already discussed. Shortly after Aschoff, Beitzke (4) recorded a similar

3

observation. He noted a low incidence of atheroma in post-mortem material in Germany after World War I; he also attrib-uted this to the effects of dietary restrictions. Other studies of patients with chronic wasting disorders who have undergone a terminal loss of weight claimed to show a reduction of arterial atheroma (5). However, not all authors were able to relate the state of nutrition to the degree of atheroma in the vessels: Winter et al. (6) found no relationship.

Eeg-Larsen (7) discussed dietary trends in Norway from 1914 to 1964 noting, in particular, the active interest in nutrition and diet, which was generated by poverty, unemployment, and the ignorance of the times. At that time certain foods such as milk, cheese, eggs, liver, and fats were designated as desirable protective features of the diet. This resulted in an increased intake of dietary calories from fat to a level of 40 percent from the previous 25 percent. He considered that the fivefold increase in the incidence of myocardial infarction from 1950 to 1964 was due to this change of diet. Here again the problem arises that better living conditions are not reflected only by a change of diet so that other factors might be involved to explain the increased incidence of infarction. Other views come from a study of chronic wasting diseases.

The relationship between degrees of atherosclerosis and ma-lignant disease has been a controversial topic for years. Some say that there is less and others that there is more arterial dis-ease in these people. The subject has been well reviewed re-cently (8 and 9), and the controversy persists. A recent detailed study of the cerebral vessels of nearly 4,000 subjects, at autopsy, has revealed a significantly lower incidence of cerebral vascular disease in subjects with malignant disorders (9). Furthermore, the relationship appeared to be independent of the site or type of malignant disease and of the presence or absence of hyper-tension, coronary atherosclerosis, cerebral vascular disease, and diabetes mellitus. Clues to a mechanism of reversing atheroscle-rosis may arise from observations of this sort, though at present the significance remains obscure and the authors take pains to point this out. A recent study from Russia found no influence of malignant disease on the degree of coronary atherosclerosis (10).

There is evidence from other studies of human autopsy material that atherosclerosis might be preventable or reversible; these have been reviewed by Strong (11). He emphasises the wide variability in the extent and severity of atherosclerosis in homogeneous human populations as one indicator. Another is the variability of the disease between different ethnic groups such as black and white and the same ethnic group in different geographical locations. Genetic differences in susceptibility can be involved to explain some of these differences. However, the clear association that has emerged between the incidence of ischaemic heart disease and certain risk factors reinforces the view that atherosclerosis is preventable, to some extent reversible.

In the 1970 Lyman Duff Memorial Lecture to the American Heart Association, Louis Katz stated, "I wish to emphasise that atherosclerosis is reversible to some extent . . . . it is not inevitable and merely a non-reversible association of aging" (12). He based this statement on epidemiological studies and animal experiments that he had made in collaboration with Stamler, Pick, Dauber, and others (13). Ruth Pick has continued this work, which will be discussed in a later chapter. Katz emphasised the importance of primary prevention of the disease and discussed the various risk factors that should be eliminated. He concluded that dietary control, suppression of smoking, and the control of hypertension were the primary prongs of preventative attack. In the past, attempts to reduce arterial atheroma by this means have often been disappointing. Knight et al. (14) was only able to cause some regression of coronary disease in three out of twenty-two patients with hypercholesterolemia who had been treated by a surgical ileal bypass despite the fact that cholesterol concentration fell by about 40 percent. Poor results of this sort are often due to the presence of advanced disease in old subjects. If, however, younger and even symptomless persons are studied, the results can be improved. Barndt et al. (15) studied femoral arteriograms of twenty-five patients all with hyperlipidemia. They ranged in age from twenty-two to sixty-five, and sixteen had no symptoms. Treatment with diet, hypolipidaemic, and, where indicated, hypotensive drugs caused regression of lesions in nine patients. These nine pa-

tients had a significant fall in blood cholesterol whereas the rest
had no such change; of these, thirteen progressed and three
showed no progress either way. This is an important piece of
work, which strongly supports Katz's early prophecy that atherosclerosis might be, at least in part, reversible.

We shall discuss later the many experiments that have shown
regression of atherosclerosis in animals when atherogenic stimuli are withdrawn. However, the ultimate proof of regression
must be demonstrated in man himself. This proof largely depends on improvements in methods for the accurate assessment
of the degree and extent of atherosclerosis in arteries. Such
methods are being developed steadily, and a subsequent chapter
will deal with the question of measurement of atheroma.

Criticism of previous studies in man that purport to show
regression of atherosclerosis rests largely on lack of precise
definition of the disease under consideration (16). Although the
prime basis of ischaemic heart disease is coronary atherosclerosis, other lesions are involved, in particular superimposed
thrombosis or even spasm of the diseased artery. Occasionally,
platelet microthrombi contribute to the ischaemic event, and
these cannot be detected save by microscopy (17). At the present
time, animal models remain the principal source of evidence
about regression, yet in no field of experimental pathology has
there been more scepticism about their use (18). The two basic
problems seem to lie with the precise definition of an atherosclerotic lesion and the acceptance of an animal that can be
matched with man. Some insist that the only acceptable lesions
are fully developed atheroma with its associated complications
of mural haemorrhage, thrombosis, and so on. Others demand
experiments in nonhuman primates and exclude all other
animal experiments from a discussion of the problem.

There is even argument about the earlier stages of the disease;
some insist that fatty streaks and spots are not early evidence of
atherosclerosis because they occur in parts of the vascular
system where later, more complex, atheroma is not found (19).
Yet the fact that fatty streaks are often found above the aortic
cusps and in the thoracic aorta whereas more advanced disease
predominates in the abdominal aorta suggests that fatty streaks
might regress. This is perhaps due to changing haemody-

namics with growth and age. Furthermore, transitions can often be found between fatty streaks and later lesions, such as fibrous plaques. A common site for this transition is within the carotid sinus area of the internal carotid artery.

There is a real need to define the basic pathophysiology of the atherosclerotic process. Many hold the view that changed endothelial permeability is the initiating event and that subsequent intimal damage may be due to the insudation of various plasma constituents followed by a proliferative repair by cells of smooth-muscle type. Using this hypothesis, one can review the source, metabolism, and effects of various constituents of the lesion and consider the likelihood that some of the constituents might not only enter but also leave the vessel wall.

References

1. Aschoff, L.: *Lectures in Pathology.* New York, Hoeber, 1924.
2. Katz, L. N., Stamler, J., and Pick, R.: *Nutrition and Atherosclerosis.* Philadelphia, Lea and Febiger, 1958.
3. Chaikoff, I. L., Nichols, C. W., Gaffey, W., and Lindsay, S.: The effect of dietary protein level on the development of naturally occurring aortic arteriosclerosis in the chicken. *J Atheroscler Res, 1:*461, 1961.
4. Beitzke, H.: Zur Entstehung der Atherosclerose, *Virchows Arch Path Anat, 267:*625, 1928.
5. Wilens, S. L.: Bearing of general nutritional state on atherosclerosis. *Arch Intern Med, 79:*129, 1947.
6. Winter, M. O., Jr., Sayre, G. P., Millikan, C. H., and Barker, N. W.: Relationship of degree of atherosclerosis of internal carotid system in the brain of women to age and coronary atherosclerosis. *Circulation, 18:*7, 1958.
7. Eeg-Larsen, N.: Dietary trends in Norway during the last fifty years. *Bibl Nutr Dieta, 6:*82, 1964.
8. Wissler, R. W. and Vesselinovitch, D.: Studies of regression of advanced atherosclerosis in experimental animals and man. *Ann NY Acad Sci, 275:*363, 1976.
9. Klassen, A. C., Loewenson, R. B., and Resch, J. A.: Cerebral atherosclerosis in selected chronic disease states. *Atherosclerosis, 18:*321, 1973.
10. Vihert, A. M., Zhoanov, V. S., and Matova, E. E.: Atherosclerosis of the aorta and coronary vessels of the heart in cases of various diseases. *J Atheroscler Res, 9:*179, 1969.
11. Strong, J. P.: Atherosclerosis, A Preventable Disease? Autopsy Evidence: International Symposium: State of Prevention and Therapy in Human

Arteriosclerosis and in Animal Models, 1977 (to be published).

12. Katz, L. N.: *Has Knowledge of Atherosclerosis Advanced Sufficiently to Warrant its Application to a Practical Prevention Program?* The 1970 Lyman Duff Memorial Lecture, Council on Arteriosclerosis, American Heart Association.

13, Stamler, J.: In Sandler, M. and Bourne, G. H. (Eds.): *Atherosclerosis and its Origins.* New York, Acad Pr, 1963, p. 231.

14. Knight, L., Scheibel, R., Amplatz, K., Varco, R. L., and Buchwald, H.: Radiographic appraisal of the Minnesota Partial Ileal Bypass Study. *Surg Forum, 23:*141, 1972.

15. Barndt, R., Blankenhorn, D. H., Crawford, D. W., and Brooks, S. H.: Regression and progression of early femoral atherosclerosis in treated hyperlipoproteinemic patients. *Ann Intern Med, 86:*139, 1977.

16. Regression of atheroma. *Br Med J, ii:*1, 1977.

17. Haerem, J. W.: Mural platelet microthrombi in sudden coronary death. *Atherosclerosis, 19:*529, 1974.

18. Progression and regression of atherosclerosis. *Br Med J, i:*481, 1976.

19. Mitchell, J. R. A. and Schwartz, C. J.: *Arterial Disease.* Oxford, Blackwell, 1965.

CHAPTER 2

COMPONENTS OF THE ATHEROSCLEROTIC LESION AND THEIR ROLE IN ATHEROGENESIS

The Vessel Wall

IN some respects, the arterial wall of large animals is structurally prone to develop arterial disease. The strange paradox is that the very structure that conducts blood to nourish various tissues is itself poorly supplied with blood. Furthermore, changes take place with increasing age that make the situation worse. For example, the aorta increases gradually in thickness after birth, and different events occur in the thoracic and abdominal aorta (1). Increased thickness of the thoracic aorta is caused by an actual increase in the numbers of lamellar units, whereas the abdominal vessel thickens by an increase in the thickness of existing lamellar units. These units consist of smooth muscle cells attached to coarse elastic fibres with surrounding bundles of collagen in a matrix of mucopolysaccharide. In other words, there is hyperplasia of units in the thoracic part and hypertrophy in the abdominal part.

This situation means increased unit tension in the abdominal aorta as compared to the thoracic. In addition, these units have a relatively poorer blood supply than the thoracic elements. The requirement that a bigger unit should develop higher tension while retaining the same blood supply is clearly a predisposing factor to hypoxia. Unlike most other mammals, the entire thickness of the human abdominal aorta is without vasa vasorum. In other large mammals it is only the inner zone of the vessel that has no blood vessels.

Even in the rabbit there is evidence of a low oxygen tension in the inner abdominal aortic media. Measurements of transmural oxygen tensions revealed an adventitial PO_2 of 27 mm Hg, an inner medial tension of 22 mm, and an intimal tension

9

of 37 mm of Hg (2). It is not surprising that hypoxic change, as may be caused by CO from cigarette smoking, is an important factor in atherogenesis.

Human arteries also become more vulnerable to hypoxia with increasing age because of progressive intimal thickening, which is present at or before birth. There is a steady accumulation of metachromatic material and collagen fibres in the intima with smooth muscle cell proliferation as well. By contrast, smooth muscle cells disappear gradually from parts of the media with replacement by mucosubstances and reticular fibres. This change is probably a reparative process, which is secondary to ischaemic death of medial muscle occasioned by the progressive intimal thickening (3).

Other workers, using polarographic methods, have shown reduced oxygen tensions in the inner parts of the arterial wall as compared to the outer parts (4), and a similar oxygen gradient has been shown across the walls of the heart (5). Thus the margin of reserve for the supply of oxygen to the arterial wall by diffusion is small. Any factors affecting this adversely are liable to lead to ischaemia and wall damage. This can occur either by an increase in metabolic activity in the vessel wall, which can be achieved by catecholamines (6), or by damage to the vasa vasorum as in diabetes mellitus or syphilis. A dramatic demonstration of the latter fact is the experimental production of medial necrosis and dissecting aneurysm when the intercostal arteries that supply the aortic vasa are tied (7).

Oxygen transport from the vascular lumen is partly dependent upon the concentrations of plasma proteins, and in most human animals these decrease with age (8). From the foregoing facts it seems that atherosclerosis in man is almost an inevitable feature of advancing age. As early as 1944, Hueper advanced the notion that hypoxia was the prime cause of the disease, leading to impaired oxidative metabolism in the vessel wall with an increase in permeability and the imbibition of plasmatic materials, which further aggravates the disease (9).

The Arterial Lipids

Lipid accumulation, mainly in the form of cholesterol and

its esters, is one of the cardinal features of occlusive atheroma. Hypoxia itself could entirely explain lipid accumulation (10), and enzymatic defects can be shown in the media of various human arteries as the intima becomes thicker. At a critical thickness of 0.15 mm, the aortic media shows a loss of oxidative enzymes in the middle part of the wall. This could lead to a reduced synthesis of lipotropic agents such as phospholipid and protein with the subsequent accumulation of cholesterol because of failure to transport it out of the vessel wall (11). In these experiments, intracellular lipid, as seen in the fatty streak, appeared before the critical intimal thickening had occurred and before medial enzyme defects had developed. Conversely, extracellular lipid was found only when intimal and medial changes could be demonstrable. Therefore, intracellular lipid accumulation is not entirely explicable in terms of hypoxia.

The appearance of lipids in the atherosclerotic plaque is susceptible to a number of explanations. It can arrive because of increased permeability of the endothelial layer or because of increased local synthesis, which may be associated with failure to transport it from the wall. Atherosclerotic lesions, in general, tend to show increased uptake of radioactively labelled carbon, but this is mainly taken into the glycerol moiety of phospholipid. The rate of uptake of labelled cholesterol is increased in atherosclerotic tissue, and the rate increases with the degree of atheroma. Furthermore, cholesterol esters are taken up directly by the diseased vessel (12). This rate of uptake is closely related to the level of plasma cholesterol so that it might be anticipated that lowering cholesterol levels might be a potent means of preventing or reversing atherosclerosis. Certainly, authors up to the present have been unable to demonstrate synthesis of cholesterol from acetate by atherosclerotic human coronary arteries (13). We shall describe experiments to support this contention in a subsequent chapter.

A considerable amount of interest has centred on the relation of low-density lipoproteins (LDL) in plasma and in the arterial wall in relationship to atherogenesis. These proteins, in common with many plasma constituents, can be demonstrated in the arterial intima (14), and they increase in quality with advancing age. Some of these lipoproteins can be readily extracted from the intima. Others are fixed in position around fibrous deposits in the vessel wall and cannot readily be re- moved. Various methods have been used to show the presence of lipoproteins, and they have been demonstrated by immuno- diffusion techniques on fluid extracted directly from the vessel wall (15).

Low-density lipoproteins in the vessel wall do exchange slowly with plasma LDL, but the rate of exchange is slow in comparison with that in the liver and spleen.

Furthermore, once cholesterol has become disassociated from its lipoprotein vehicle, it becomes inaccessible to intracellular metabolic process and steadily accumulates in the arterial wall (16). Reversibility of the lipid component of the lesion, there- fore, is likely to involve the lipids near the surface of the lesion that have gained entry recently (17).

Many workers have shown that the physicochemical form in which cholesterol is present in the tissue determines whether it can readily be removed. Byers and Friedman (18) studied the effect of intra-aortic and intraperitoneal insertion of cholesterol esters. When cholesterol-acetate was implanted as a solid cyl- inder, the cholesterol remained undissolved. If the same ester was injected in a finely dispersed state, it was taken up by abundant macrophages and was retained in the tissue. If the cholesterol was injected in a lipoprotein vehicle, it was re- moved rapidly from the tissues. Adams and Morgan (19) found that cholesterol, implanted subcutaneously, rapidly disap- peared from the tissues when highly unsaturated phosphatidyl choline was injected with it. They suggested that this resulted in the formation of cholesteryl arachidonate, which was the least sclerogenic of thirteen esters of cholesterol that they had tested previously.

This work suggests that the ease with which cholesterol emerges from a tissue will depend not only on its physical form but also upon the type of fatty acid with which it is esterified. Necrosis of tissue leading to a lack of phagocytic cells in the vicinity of the lipid material is another factor that may hinder removal. There are many factors that contribute to necrosis in atherosclerotic plaques. We have already indicated that hypoxia may play a part. In addition, the nature of the lipid is also important, some forms being more necrogenic than others. For example, tissue implants of 26-hydroxycholesterol and other forms lead to extensive necrosis (20).

Regression of such lipid-laden, necrotic areas of the lesion can only be accomplished by phagocytic cells; a number of workers have emphasised the important role of macrophages in the atherosclerotic process. Day (21) reviewed the situation in 1964, making the point that the cells that phagocytose and remove lipid through the endothelial surface may also be concerned in lipid synthesis and deposition.

Adams (22) summarised evidence that lipids are resorbed more rapidly when phagocytic macrophages are present. Atheromatous lesions with few phagocytes lose their lipid component slowly when regressive measures are applied. Xanthomas of the skin, however, can be induced to lose lipid rapidly, and they are rich in phagocytic cells.

Arterial Mucopolysaccharides

Acid mucopolysaccharides form another group of extracellular materials that are found in the arterial wall in atherosclerotic disease. Their role in atherogenesis and their significance in terms of potential regression of lesions require discussion. Mucopolysaccharides (MPS) can be found in the intima and media of normal and diseased aortas, and there is considerable confusion in the literature because, quite often, the particular type of MPS is not clearly stated. For example, chondroitin sulphate C in the young intima may be a normal phenomenon associated with the presence of fine collagen fibres in the intima. In addition, the MPS have many other roles in the vessel wall. They have variously been assigned mechanical and structural properties, involvement in repair and calcification, and are also implicated in anticoagulation and lipid clearance (23) (24).

The diverse potential roles of mucosubstances in the arterial wall make it likely that they have something to do with atherogenesis and that attempts to remove or alter their composition might yield fruitful results in studies on regression of atherosclerotic disease. Mast cells are a principle source of mucopolysaccharides in tissues; the relationships between mast cell numbers, amounts of mucosubstances, and degrees of atherosclerosis have been the subject of much study. Cairns and Constantinides (25) actually suggested that the number of mast cells was less in the myocardium of patients with coronary atheroma than in the normal heart, and Paterson and Mills (26) found no relation between mast cell numbers and severity of atheroma. However, many other authors have described increased numbers of mast cells in the adventitia of vessels affected by atherosclerosis [Hjelman (27), Sundberg (28), Pollak (29) and Pomerance (30)]. Poucher et al. (31) studied the number of mast cells throughout the arterial wall in different stages of atherosclerosis. There were more mast cells in the adventitia than elsewhere in the vessel wall, and they were found around vasa vasorum and nerves. The number in the adventitia was greatest where intimal atherosclerotic thickening was most evident. The authors attribute the small numbers of intimal mast cells, in these areas, to disintegration of the cells as the atherosclerotic process develops as well as the possibility that some of these cells become converted to fibrocytes. The general theme of their argument is that mast cells provoke an inflammatory response in the arterial wall by providing ground substances such as hyaluronic acid and also by liberating heparin, which provokes connective tissue proliferation (32).

The Inflammatory Component

Few workers have much to say about the inflammatory component of the atherosclerotic lesion, yet inflammatory cells are commonly seen either within the lesion itself or in the adjacent adventitia. This inflammatory component is of increasing importance in view of the suggestion that atherosclerosis is essentially a proliferative response to intimal injury (33) and the more recent suggestion that atherosclerotic plaques are initially monoclonal in origin and, hence, could be caused by injurious agents such as viruses (34).

Restrepo and Tracy (35) studied degrees of focal necrosis and leucocytic infiltration in fatty streaks and were able to show that the severity of these two components was related to the degree of elevation of the lesion. This suggested, to them, that the presence of inflammatory components in the intimal lesions could be related to their tendency to progress and narrow the lumen of the vessel. McCullagh and Page (36) emphasise the importance of collagen as an occlusive factor in the atherosclerotic artery. Experiments in dogs revealed a specific five to twenty times increase in collagen synthesis in the atherosclerotic parts of arteries from these animals (37). They were also able to demonstrate an inhibitory effect on collagen synthesis of cis hydroxyproline in aortic slices taken from the dogs and grown in tissue culture. Clearly, then, the inflammatory components of the atherosclerotic lesion, whether they be mucopolysaccharides, inflammatory cells or collagen, must be considered carefully in deliberations concerning the possible prevention or attempted regression of atherosclerotic arterial disease since they can contribute to vascular narrowing.

A lot has been written about the role of vascular calcification both in atherogenesis and as a complication of the process. At the present time, calcification is not regarded either as a cause or as an important complication of atherosclerosis and need not be discussed further in relation to regression (38).

Arterial Endothelium

Many workers now accept the view that the prime event in the initiation of the atherosclerotic plaque is direct injury to the endothelial sheet, which then leads to increased vascular permeability and the entry of damaging substances such as certain lipoproteins. There is, however, a good deal of debate over the precise way in which the endothelial sheet is injured, and it is appropriate to review some of the hypotheses here as they relate to possible mechanisms for prevention and regression of atherosclerotic disease. We have already discussed the inflammatory component of atheroma, and there are some (39) who proposed that atherogenesis is the result of such a reaction on the vessel surface. They propose that an antigen or antibody reaction, possibly caused by an infectious agent, triggers the complement system. This is an easily activated complex of biologically aggressive compounds that may damage endothelial cells. Complement can increase in amount in the serum during or after an infectious disease. Alternatively, an increase in macromolecules derived from diet or aggregates of antigen-antibody complexes may activate the system and lead to increased endothelial permeability. An uneven distribution of such macromolecules due to turbulence in the blood at branches or divisions in vessels could account for the uneven distribution of vascular damage and subsequent atheroma. This is an ingenious notion meriting serious consideration because it draws together a number of factors that have recently been implicated as atherogenic agents.

Studies of the endothelial sheet lining blood vessels have been done in a number of ways. Considerable confusion arose initially because of poor technical methods. A proper view of the endothelial sheet is now possible using scanning electron microscopy with the adjunct of silver staining to reveal the intercellular junctions and by fixing vessels at physiological pressure, which prevents collapse of the vessel and buckling of the endothelial sheet (40).

Other studies have shown multiple pinocytotic vesicles on both the intimal and luminal side of endothelial cells, and these are the main mechanism for transport of materials into the vascular wall. The normal intercellular junctions are tight without pores in the normal vessel. Electron microscopic and fluorescent antibody techniques have also shown that endothelial cells contain contractile proteins similar to platelet thrombosthenin and smooth muscle actomyosin (41). Much debate surrounds the relationship of endothelial cells to others in the normal and atherosclerotic vessel wall. For example, the origin of smooth muscle cells that come to line vascular prostheses is still obscure. Some say that they derive from circulating cells in the blood, and others hold the view that they might be modified endothelial cells and that smooth muscle cells and endothelial cells derive from a common ancestor in the vessel wall.

A useful technique for studying endothelial permeability is the administration of Evans blue intravenously. This device was well known to Anitschkow and has been used by several workers since the early part of this century. Basically, it depends upon the fact that the dye binds itself to plasma albumen; if parts of the vessel wall take up the dye, it means that these parts are points of increased permeability to the plasma protein. When the dye is given to a normal animal, such as a baboon, focal points of staining of the intima of vessel can be faintly discerned. These points of staining are often situated distal to branches in a vessel such as the thoracic aorta and correspond with points of turbulence and more than normal stress in the vessel wall. When the blood pressure rises, the entry of Evans blue is increased. This is thought to be due not merely to an increase of perfusion pressure but also to stretching of the aortic wall and has been supported by experiments on aortic strips studied *in vitro* (42). Other parameters of endothelial sheet function have been studied under various experimentally induced circumstances. H. Payling Wright (43) studied the uptake of tritiated thymidine by endothelial cells to see if mitoses were evenly scattered through the sheet of cells. Using the aorta of the guinea pig and subsequently making Häutchen preparations that could be viewed *en face*, she was able to show that mitoses were not related to the age of the animal and also that they occurred more often in the proximal than in the distal aorta. This relates to the work of authors who showed that the degree of stretching in the aortic wall was greater in the proximal than in the distal part of the vessel. Increased permeability and increased mitoses are, therefore, related in the proximal aorta. However, atherosclerosis is often more severe in the abdominal than in the thoracic aorta so that it is difficult to know what these changes in permeability and cell turnover mean in relation to atherogenesis.

Schwartz and his colleagues have done a number of experiments with pigs, and they and other workers have related focal areas of uptake of Evans blue to increased uptake of tritiated thymidine (44). These focal areas also have an increased turnover of free cholesterol in the inner part of the vessel wall, increased permeability to fibrinogen, and so on.

Hypertension injures the inner vessel wall; there is little doubt about this and of the part that it plays in atherogenesis. Indeed, one of the most potent ways available to us in the prevention and possible reversal of atherosclerosis is the early control of hypertension. It is not surprising that lowering of blood pressure in middle age has little effect upon the results of coronary atherosclerosis. The disease is often too well established by that time.

Apart from hypertension, hyperlipidaemia is also a well-recognized aggravating atherogenic factor. However, it is not clear whether the hyperlipidaemia is a prime damaging agent to the endothelial sheet or whether it produces a secondary occlusive effect by aggravating lipid accumulation in the damaged arterial wall. Silkworth et al. (45) examined aortic endothelium, by the Häutchen technique, from rabbits fed on a cholesterol-enriched diet for varying lengths of time. They found an increase in stomata, multinucleate giant cells of endothelial origin, and leucocytes, particularly near to emergent branches of the aorta. Other workers have found that hypercholesterolemia induces an increased number of mitoses and increased DNA synthesis in endothelial cells, leading to increased permeability that might provide a substrate for subsequent atherosclerosis (46).

Before accepting such results at their face value, however, it is important to remember that much of the experimental work is done with diets containing commercial cholesterol. It has recently been shown that such cholesterol is not pure and that methanol extracts made from it have a selective angiotoxic effect, which is independent of the cholesterol itself (47).

Bonders and Björkerud, in a series of papers, have attempted to clarify the role of endothelial damage and the causes of endothelial damage as potential atherogenic factors. In 1975 (48), they studied the uptake of free and esterified cholesterol by aortic endothelium in live rabbits. Where the endothelium was intact, they found a direct relationship between the uptake of labelled free and esterified cholesterol in the ratio of 20:1. This suggested to them that the process involved was one of active transport and that hydrolysis of cholesterol ester was a primary step in it. On the other hand, where the endothelium was defective, they showed that the cholesterol content of the defective area was higher than in the intact area and that the uptake of free and esterified cholesterol was also higher. This suggested filtration of lipoproteins in the zone of defective endothelium.

Previously (49), the same authors had studied the types of cholesteryl esters in plasma and in the arterial wall after the induction of atherosclerotic lesions by mechanical injury. They found that plasma cholesteryl esters contained a majority of diunsaturated fatty acids, whereas monounsaturated acids were the predominant esterifying agent in the arterial wall itself. If the arterial wall was allowed to repair itself, the proportion of polyunsaturated fatty acids increased. This is an important observation in relation to regression because it suggested that hydrolysis of cholesteryl esters, in the arterial wall, might be an essential prerequisite for the elimination of cholesterol deposits from the atheromatous plaque.

Not everyone would agree that the atherosclerotic process is necessarily the result of a single injury to one compartment of the vessel wall such as, for example, the endothelium. It is possible that simultaneous events take place in atherogenesis, involving several components in the reaction. The series of events that follow a longitudinal intimal injury to the rabbit aorta illustrates this point. The early change is one of necrosis and infiltration by leucocytes; a foreign body reaction follows with ingrowth of new capillaries into the area of tissue damage. Tiny thrombi form on the surface, and re-endothelialisation follows quickly. At the same time, the vessel dilates due to damage of the adjacent smooth muscle (50). The same workers (51) found evidence of damaged endothelium and of adjacent medial smooth muscle in the aortas of normal rabbits and rats. These areas of damage were found at branches and in other areas of increased haemodynamic strain. This suggests that even the normal aorta is preconditioned to develop atherosclerosis. However, neither the rabbit nor the rat ordinarily develop atherosclerotic disease without provocation of some sort so that possible programmes for prevention and regression should not be hindered by the supposed inevitability of atherosclerotic disease, which these studies have suggested.

Arterial Smooth Muscle

Views about the type of cell that is predominantly involved

in the early phases of the atherosclerotic process have changed considerably over the years and continue to do so. Geer and Haust (41) have reviewed the matter extensively in their excellent monograph, and more recent studies are contained in the volume by Schettler and Weizel (2). The issue centres, at the moment, on the role of those cells that have the structural features of smooth muscle. The features are not sharply defined, as they tend to vary with the age of the animal and also with the stage of the atherosclerotic process. For this reason, terms such as *myointimal cells* have come into use. There is no doubt that some cells in the intimal lesion have the characteristics of smooth muscle. They show the usually acceptable criteria of a well-defined basement membrane, numerous pinocytotic vesicles along the plasma membrane, and an abundance of cytoplasmic myofilaments. But other cells occur alongside these, and their precise relationship to smooth muscle remains debatable. It is important to emphasise the lack of precise definition.

Some (52) have described intimal lesions that are entirely composed of smooth muscle and do not contain lipid and infer that these are the early stages of atherosclerosis, with degenerative changes such as lipid accumulation coming later in the process. By contrast, Wissler (53) concedes the presence of one cell type in the process but regards it as a multifunctional cell that can develop and initiate a variety of processes according to the stimulus it might receive. At that time, in 1968, he posed a number of important questions, some of which have a solution; many do not. We still do not know why this multipurpose cell is deflected from its prime role of elastin synthesis to that of collagen and mucopolysaccharide production, why the cells proliferate and, if they do so, migrate from media to intima. Much remains to be learned about the basic biochemistry of these cells. It is known that impairment of cross-linkage in collagen and elastin, which can be induced by administering β-aminopropionitrile to young animals, does result in increased synthesis of acid mucopolysaccharide in the arterial wall accompanied by hypertrophy of smooth muscle cells (54). Similar effects can be seen in deficiency of vitamin B_6 (pyridoxine). Recent work has suggested that the arteriosclerotic effect of B_6

deficiency (55) may be related to increased use of homocystine and failure of cystathione formation from homocysteine. If sulphur-containing amino acids are fed to animals, they produce atherosclerosis; they are more potent than lipids in this respect in that they produce larger lesions earlier (56). The precise role of homocysteine in promoting the growth of cells and intercellular matrix in the vessel wall is largely undetermined and provides yet another avenue in the possible route to the prevention of atherosclerosis.

Homocysteinuria is a rare disease in man but has a well-known association with the development of premature arterial disease. If homocysteine is given intravenously to baboons, the effect is to cause areas of endothelial damage with extensive platelet aggregation on the damaged areas. Adjacent smooth muscle cells proliferate rapidly, and an atherosclerotic lesion appears. While this cellular proliferation might be entirely due to homocysteine itself, another agent has been shown to be present. Ross (57) has shown a platelet-dependent factor that causes smooth muscle cell proliferation. This can be shown by tissue culture methods. This sort of observation raises the fundamental question about the role of blood constituents in the atherogenic process and particularly highlights the possible activity of blood platelets.

Blood Coagulation and Atherogenesis

The haemostatic role of the blood platelets has never been in doubt, but the possible contribution that it and other components of the coagulation mechanism make to the atherosclerotic lesions has been debated ever since Rokitinsky conceived the incrustation hypothesis in the middle of the nineteenth century. Much has been learned about platelets in recent years, and a good deal of this new information has recreated the view that the cells might play an important role in atherogenesis (33). Platelets are active contractile cells that contain a variety of amines that can alter the permeability of the vessel wall and also contain substances such as the smooth muscle stimulating factor. The burning issue is whether platelets can adhere to the normal vessel wall and initiate atherosclerosis. Not that this needs postulating, however, as we have already discussed experiments that show loss of endothelium in parts of vessels where branches occur (48, 51). In 1964, Mustard et al. reviewed the problem extensively and concluded that evidence implicating the accretion of blood elements in the development of atherosclerosis was established. At that time they emphasised the need to determine the stage of the disease at which they started to operate. A wide range of drugs alters platelet activity *in vitro*. It is more difficult to affect their function *in vivo*. Even if this could be done successfully and relatively early in the life of the human subject, it is still not clear what effect such a regime might have on atherogenesis.

There is, however, a small group of cases of coronary artery obstruction where attempts to reduce platelet aggregation might be advantageous. These are persons who die suddenly and unexpectedly and yet have no major occlusive lesion in the epicardial cornary arteries. In these subjects, extensive platelet plugging of small intramyocardial vessels has been demonstrated (59). A similar fatal condition has been induced in swine by the injection of adenosine diphosphate into the coronary arteries. This is a potent aggregator of platelets and leads to widespread plugging of small coronary vessels and myocardial infarction (60).

It may be that platelet aggregation plays an important role in causing sudden death in patients who have established coronary artery disease as well (61). Enough is not known about this because few workers have attempted a detailed survey of cardiac arteries for the presence of such aggregates and also because platelet aggregates are not easy to define by conventional staining methods, particularly if the arteries have already been opened at necropsy. It is, nevertheless, an important matter to resolve when considering prevention of the end point of atherosclerotic heart disease, which is often sudden unexpected death.

Other components of the clotting mechanism have been demonstrated in the vessel wall using empirical staining, immunofluorescence, and chemical analysis. Extensive studies by Elsbeth Smith and her colleagues (62) have shown the presence of fibrinogen and fibrin in the vessel wall. Indeed, with the possible exception of very low density lipoprotein, all plasma proteins that have been sought have been found in the intima. The system is a complex one in developing lesions where high concentrations of plasma constituents are present. Not only is the ordinary process of the conversion of fibrinogen to fibrin and its subsequent degradation by plasma taking place, in addition, some of the fibrin degradation products may inhibit clotting, and some fragments of low molecular weight may cause an increased permeability of the vessel wall, leading to the contraction of smooth muscle as well (63).

Not only were fibrinogen and fibrin present in lesions, but Smith et al. (62) found that 2 percent of the tissue dry weight of normal intima contained fibrinogen and fibrin in the ratio of 1:0 to 1:5. In the early lesions, the proportion of fibrinogen and low-density lipoprotein was increased. Others (64) have shown similar deposits in slight degrees of intimal thickening in coronary arteries; these authors have invoked the early involvement of blood coagulation substances in atherogenesis. The problem remains unsolved, but it is salutary to consider that severe coronary atherosclerosis and thrombosis are almost exclusive to man. In practically all other animals, coronary atherosclerosis is rare and coronary thrombosis most unusual in relation to it. It is difficult to escape a relationship between the two processes. It may just be that severe ulcerative atheroma leads to thrombosis, but it is equally possible that the thrombotic process is the initiator of atherogenesis.

Summary

In this chapter we have brought together the main performers on the atherogenic stage. The next step is to examine the risk factors to see how they might be modified and to study the effects of such modifications, mainly in experimental animals.

References

1. Wolinsky, H. and Glagov, S.: Comparison of abdominal and thoracic aortic medial structure in mammals. Deviation of man from the usual

pattern. *Circ Res, 25:*677, 1969.
2. Niinikoski, J., Heughan, C., and Hunt, T. K.: Oxygen tensions in the aortic wall of normal rabbits. *Atherosclerosis, 17:*353, 1973.
3. Lopes de Faria, J.: Role of wall factors in the pathogenesis of coronary atherosclerosis. *J Atheroscler Res, 8:*291, 1968.
4. Moss, A. J., Samuelson, P., Angell, C., and Minken, S. L.: Polarographic evaluation of transmural oxygen availability in intact muscular arteries. *J Atheroscler Res, 8:*803, 1968.
5. Moss, A. J.: Intramyocardial oxygen tension. *Cardiovasc Res, 2:*314, 1968.
6. Kosan, R. L. and Burton, A.: Oxygen consumption of arterial smooth muscle as a function of active tone and passive stretch. *Circ Res, 18:*79, 1966.
7. Wilens, S. L., Malcolm, J. A., and Vasquez, J. M.: Experimental infarction (medial necrosis) of the dog's aorta. *Am J Pathol, 47:*695, 1965.
8. Chisolm, G. M., Gainer, J. L., Stoner, G. E., and Gainer, J. V.: Plasma proteins, oxygen transport and atherosclerosis. *Atherosclerosis, 15:*327, 1972.
9. Hueper, W. C.: Arteriosclerosis. The anoxemia theory. *Arch Pathol, 39:*162, 245, 350, 1944.
10. Dixon, K. C.: Deposition of globular lipid in arterial cells in relation to anoxia. *Am J Pathol, 39:*65, 1961.
11. Adams, C. W. M. and Bayliss, O. B.: The relationship between diffuse intimal thickening, medial enzyme failure and intimal lipid deposition in various human arteries. *J Atheroscler Res, 10:*327, 1969.
12. Bell, F. P., Lofland, H. B., Jr., and Stokes, N. A.: Cholesterol flux in vitro in aortas of cholesterol-fed and non-cholesterol-fed pigeons. *Atherosclerosis, 11:*235, 1970.
13. Hashimoto, H., Tillmanns, H., Sarma, J. S. M., Mao, J., Holden, E., and Bing, R. J.: Lipid metabolism in human nonatherosclerotic coronary arteries and saphenous veins. *Atherosclerosis, 19:*35, 1974.
14. Smith, E. B. and Slater, R.: The chemical and immunological assay of low density lipoproteins extracted from human aortic intima. *Atherosclerosis, 11:*417, 1970.
15. Klimov, A. N., Denisenko, A. D., and Magracheva, E. Y. A.: Preparation of tissue fluid of the vessel wall and deterioration of its lipoproteins. *Atherosclerosis, 19:*243, 1974.
16. Scott, P. J., and Hurley, P. J.: The distribution of radio-iodinated serum albumen and low-density lipoprotein in tissues and the arterial wall. *Atherosclerosis, 11:*77, 1970.
17. Adams, C. W. M.: Tissue changes and lipid entry in developing atheroma.
18. Byers, S. O. and Friedman, M.: Tissue reactions to forms of cholesterol. *Arch Pathol, 76:*553, 1963.
19. Adams, C. W. M. and Morgan, R. S.: The effect of saturated and

polyunsaturated lecithins on the resorbtion of 4–¹⁴C cholesterol from subcutaneous implants. *J Pathol, 94:*73, 1967.

20. Harland, W. A., Smith, A. G., and Gilbert, J. D.: Tissue reaction to atheroma lipids. *J Pathol, 111:*247, 1973.
21. Day, A. J.: The macrophage system, lipid metabolism and atherosclerosis. *J Atheroscler Res, 4:*117, 1964.
22. Adams, C. W. M., Bayliss, O. B., and Turner, D. R.: Phagocytes, lipid-removal and regression of atheroma. *J Pathol, 116:*225, 1975.
23. Kumar, V., Berenson, G. S., Ruiz, H., Dalferes, E. R., and Strong, J. P.: Acid mucopolysacharrides of human aorta. Part 1 — Variations with maturation. *J Atheroscler Res, 7:*573, 1967.
24. Kumar, V. Berenson, G. S., Ruiz, H., Dalferes, E. R., and Strong, J. P.: Acid mucopolysacharrides of human aorta. Part 2 — Variations with atherosclerotic involvement. *J Atheroscler Res, 7:*583, 1967.
25. Cairns, A. and Constantinides, P.: Mast cells in human atherosclerosis. *Science, 120:*31, 1954.
26. Paterson, J. C. and Mills, J.: Myocardial mast cell counts in coronary sclerosis. *Arch Pathol, 66:*335, 1958.
27. Hjelmman, G. and Wegelius, O.: *Soc Sci Fennica Commentationes Biol, 15:*6, 1954.
28. Sundberg, M.: On the mast cells in the human vascular wall. A quantitative study on changes at different ages. *Acta Pathol Microbiol Scand (Suppl), 107,* 1955.
29. Pollak, O. J.: Mast cells in the circulatory system of man. *Circulation, 16:*1084, 1957.
30. Pomerance, A.: Peri-arterial mast cells in coronary atheroma and thrombosis. *J Pathol Bacteriol, 76:*55, 1958.
31. Pouchlev, A., Youroukova, K., and Kiprov, D.: Changes in the number of mast cells in the human arterial wall. *J Atheroscler Res, 6:*342, 1966.
32. Bensley, S. H.: Histological studies of the reactions of cells and intercellular substances of loose connective tissue to the spreading factor of testicular extracts. *Ann NY Acad Sci, 52:*983, 1950.
33. Gresham, G. A.: Early events in atherogenesis. *Lancet, i:*614, 1975.
34. Benditt, E. P. and Benditt, J. M.: Evidence for a monoclonal origin of human atherosclerotic plaques. *Proc Natl Acad Sci USA, 70:*1753, 1973.
35. Restrepo, P. and Tracy, R. E.: Variations in human aortic fatty streaks among geographic locations. *Atherosclerosis, 21:*179, 1975.
36. McCullagh, K. G. and Page, I. H.: In Schettler, G. and Weizel, A.: Increased collagen synthesis in early rabbit atherosclerosis and its inhibition by cis-hydroxyproline in atherosclerosis, 3rd ed. Berlin, Springer-Verlag, 1974, p. 239.
37. McCullagh, K. G. and Ehrhart, L. A.: Increased arterial collagen synthesis in experimental canine. *Atherosclerosis, 19:*13, 1974.
38. McCullagh, K. G.: Arteriosclerosis in the African elephant. *Athero-

sclerosis, 21:37, 1975.

39. Geertinger, P. and Srensen, H.: Complement and arteriosclerosis. *Atherosclerosis*, 18:65, 1973.

40. Davies, P. F., Reidy, M. A., Goode, T. B., and Bowyer, D. E.: Scanning electron microscopy in the evaluation of endothelial integrity of the fatty lesion in atherosclerosis. *Atherosclerosis*, 25:125, 1976.

41. Geer, J. C. and Haust, M. D.: *Smooth Muscle Cells in Atherosclerosis*. Monographs on Atherosclerosis, vol. 2. Basel, S. Karger, 1972, p. 30.

42. Duncan, L. E., Buck, K., Jr., and Lynch, A.: The effect of pressure and stretching on the passage of labelled albumen into canine aortic wall. *J Atheroscler Res*, 5:69, 1965.

43. Payling Wright, H.: Mitosis patterns in aortic endothelium. *Atherosclerosis*, 15:93, 1972.

44. Somer, J. B., Bell, F. P., and Schwartz, C. J.: Focal differences in lipid metabolism of the young pig aorta. *Atherosclerosis*, 20:11, 1974.

45. Silkworth, J. B., McClean, B., and Stehbens, W. E.: Aortic endothelium in hypercholesterolemia. *Atherosclerosis*, 22:335, 1975.

46. Florentin, R. A., Nam, S. C., Lee, K. T., Lee, K. J., and Thomas, W. A.: Increased mitotic activity in the aortas of swine. *Arch Pathol*, 88:463, 1969.

47. Imai, H., Lee, K. T., Taylor, C. B., and Werthessen, N. T.: Angiotoxicity of methanol-soluble fraction in altered cholesterol. *Circulation (Supp. 4)*, 48:42, 1973.

48. Bondjers, G. and Björkerud, S.: Cholesterol accumulation and content in regions with defined endothelial integrity in the normal rabbit aorta. *Atherosclerosis*, 17:71, 1973.

49. Bondjers, G. and Björkerud, S.: Arterial repair and atherosclerosis after mechanical injury (Part 4). *Atherosclerosis*, 15:273, 1972.

50. Björkerud, S. and Bondjers, G.: Arterial repair and atherosclerosis after medial injury (Part 2). *Atherosclerosis*, 14:259, 1971.

51. Björkerud, S. and Bondjers, G.: Endothelial integrity and viability in the aorta of the normal rabbit and rat as evaluated with dye exclusion tests and interference contrast microscopy. *Atherosclerosis*, 15:285, 1972.

52. Antonius, J. I. and Hill, L. D.: Smooth muscle in human occlusive arterial disease. *J Atheroscler Res*, 8:111, 1968.

53. Wissler, R. W.: The arterial medial cell, smooth muscle or multifunctional mesenchyme? *J Atheroscler Res*, 8:201, 1968.

54. Alper, R., Prior, J. T., and Ruegamer, W. R.: Histological and biochemical studies on the ground substance of the aortas of lathyritic rats. *J Atheroscler Res*, 8:787, 1968.

55. Rinehart, J. F. and Greenberg, L. D.: Arteriosclerotic lesions in pyridoxine deficient monkeys. *Am J Pathol*, 25:481, 1949.

56. McCully, K. S. and Wilson, R. B.: Homocysteine theory of arteriosclerosis. *Atherosclerosis*, 22:215, 1975.

57. Ross, R., Glomset, J., Kariya, B., Harker, L.: A platelet-dependent serum factor that stimulates the proliferation of arterial smooth muscle cells

in vitro. *Proc Nat Acad Sci USA, 71:*1207, 1974.

58. Mustard, J. F., Murphy, E. A., Rowsell, H. C., and Downie, H. G.: Platelets and atherosclerosis. *J Atheroscler Res, 4:*1, 1964.

59. Haerem, J. W.: Platelet aggregates in intra-myocardial vessels of patients dying suddenly and unexpectedly of coronary artery disease. *Atherosclerosis, 15:*199, 1972.

60. Jorgensen, L., Rowsell, H. C., Hovig, T., Glynn, M. F., and Mustard, J. F.: Adenosine diphosphate-induced platelet aggregation and myocardial infarction in swine. *Lab Invest, 17:*616, 1967.

61. Haerem, J. W.: Sudden coronary death: The occurrence of platelet aggregates in the epicardial arteries of man. *Atherosclerosis, 14:*417, 1977.

62. Smith, E. B., Alexander, K. M., and Massie, I. B.: Insoluble "fibrin" in human aortic intima. *Atherosclerosis, 23:*19, 1976.

63. Kwaan, H. C. and Barlow, G. H.: Nature and biological activities of degradation products of fibrinogen and fibrin. *Ann Rev Med, 24:*335, 1973.

64. Hudson, J. and McCaughey, W. T. E.: Mural thrombosis and atherogenesis in coronary arteries and aorta. *Atherosclerosis, 19:*543, 1974.

CHAPTER 3

ATHEROGENIC AND RISK FACTORS

Introduction

MOST human beings have fatty streaks in their aortas by the time they are ten years of age; this is true for many populations independent of their ethnic or geographical origins. By the age of twenty, raised lesions can be found in the aorta and also in the coronary arteries; the frequency and extent of these lesions run parallel to subsequent clinical manifestations of coronary artery disease. It seems, then, that the attack upon the problem of coronary artery disease must start in the young adult, and this has been emphasised by a study of New Orleans cases by Strong and McGill (1). Having taken standard sections from the same location in the coronary arteries of different subjects, they were able to show that musculoelastic intimal thickening occurred even before lipid accumulation, and they were also unable to distinguish clearly between fatty streaks and fibrous plaques. This suggested that a gradual transition was taking place. Another analysis was made of the predictive value of fatty streaks for the development of advanced lesions in middle age (2). This showed that fatty streaking was more intense in young Negros than in other comparable age groups, yet they developed less extensive advanced disease in later life. It does seem that the prevention of the conversion of fatty streaks into fibrous plaques should be the main target. Because the amount of lipid in the lesion determines its conversion to a fibrous plaque, an attack upon lipid accumulation in the arterial wall seems reasonable. There is much evidence from human and experimental animal studies to connect serum lipids, diet, atheroma, and coronary heart disease; atherosclerosis could be considered largely as a problem of nutrition (3). If this is true, the preventative programme must start early, certainly not later than the second or third decade. Lipids have always provided the central theme in thoughts about athero-

28

genesis ever since cholesterol was found to be a constituent of atherosclerotic lesions in the nineteenth century. There are other risk factors for some of which a role is clearly evident; others have been more vaguely implicated. Various reviews of such risk factors have been made, the most recent comprehensive and balanced commentary being that of Ancel Keys (4).

Epidemiology — Diet

An examination of the incidence of coronary artery disease in different races and at different times might be expected to indicate potential risk factors in certain communities. It might also be expected that changing habits in populations might be reflected in a changing incidence of coronary heart disease. Changes do occur but can easily be misinterpreted. For example, a number of studies purporting to show racial differences in the incidence of coronary heart disease were in reality not due to any inborn racial characteristic but were more closely related to diet. When the diet of such people as Javanese, Japanese, and Yemenite Jews changed to that of Western type, the incidence of coronary artery disease increased (5, 6). Perhaps the best illustration of repeated anecdotal confusion is provided by the various statements about diet and arterial disease in the primitive Eskimo. Once a detailed, accurate assessment of the situation had been made, it became clear that there was no justification for the often quoted view that Eskimos live on a high-fat diet and yet have a low incidence of coronary heart disease (7).

A study of different social classes in the United Kingdom has shown a higher incidence in Class I than in Classes IV and V. Morris et al. suggested that the lack of physical activity in persons in the higher social Class I was the principal factor and supported the view with the observation that London bus-drivers were more prone to the diet of coronary heart disease than the bus conductors (8). However, a subsequent study revealed other factors such as obesity, higher serum cholesterol, and hypertension to be more frequent in the drivers.

Epidemiology — Exercise

A possible relationship between physical activity, or lack of it, and coronary heart disease has not been clearly established. Comparisons have been made between active and less active people, but they are not strictly comparable. The question why the less active have selected themselves into that group is not often asked (5). Experimental studies on the effects of exercise on the presence of coronary heart disease are few and inconclusive. It is more appropriate to quote them here than in a later section on experimental studies of other atherogenic factors.

Weiss et al. (9) reviewed much of the experimental work up to that time. In rabbits, for example, some reports describe a reduction of lesions, others no effect, and others the production of myocardial infarction after exercise. In dogs exercise accelerated atherogenesis, whereas in rats it promoted the development of a more extensive coronary collateral circulation. Cholesterol-induced lesions in birds are said to regress on exercise; the same applies to spontaneous atherosclerosis in ducks and geese but not in cockerels or pigeons. Weiss and his colleagues (9) studied a large number of chickens in three sorts of cages. They found no evidence that restriction of movement in small cages had any effect on the incidence of spontaneous avian atherosclerosis. A later, twenty-two-month study of a small number of pigs claimed to show a reduction of atherosclerosis in the exercised animals, but the results were hardly significant (10).

It is not easy to assess the value of exercise in any prevention programme of atherosclerosis. A decrease in the incidence of myocardial infarction is evident in all who have cycled for many years (11). It would be interesting to know of any differences in patterns of mortality in those cyclists who died of other causes. Nevertheless, exercise programmes are probably of emotional, physical, and medical benefit.

Epidemiology — Behaviour Patterns

The role of stress, however that is defined, and patterns of behaviour in atherogenesis is probably one of the most hotly debated subjects in the field. It has long been held that executive responsibility causes a higher risk of coronary heart disease. However, a large study of 270,000 men in the Bell Telephone System in the United States has dispelled the idea (12). In fact, it was conclusively shown that men who had attended a university were less prone to coronary heart disease than those who had not.

Equally uncertain is the role of personality as reflected in a particular pattern of behaviour in the production of disease of the coronary arteries. Friedman and his colleagues classified men into two categories: Type A and Type B. Type A was the hard-driving individual who had a continuous battle with living. Type B was more vaguely defined and more easygoing. They were able to show a relationship between behaviour type, serum cholesterol and triglycerides, hyperinsulinism, and discharge of norepinephrine (13). Not all would agree that Type A behaviour pattern is the most important determinant of coronary heart disease. Indeed, Keith et al. were unable to confirm the relationship (14). Even if the relationship were firmly established, the question remains, can such a behaviour type be altered?

Not much experimental work has been done on the effects of psychosocial factors in atherogenesis. The principle champion in this field is H. L. Ratcliffe, who has made extensive studies. Basically, he has shown that various forms of social interaction in chickens, swine, and monkeys resulted in adrenal cortical and medullary hypertrophy accompanied by arteriosclerotic changes in the intramural branches of the coronary arteries with foci of myocardial fibrosis (15).

Risk Factors

A number of studies have been made in the United States and elsewhere to define the risk factors for coronary heart disease more accurately. Kemp et al. (16) started a programme in 1948, which ran for twenty-three years. Three predominantly important factors were identified. For example, the National Cooperative Pooling Project made the point that men aged thirty to fifty-nine were eight times more liable to develop coronary heart disease if the diastolic pressure was 90 mm Hg or more, if the serum cholesterol was greater than 250 mg/dl, and if they smoked cigarettes at all (17). Kemp et al. (18) analysed the results of various studies of men at risk and were able to eliminate degrees of physical activity, skin fold thickness (as a measure of obesity), and vital capacity as prognosticators of a tendency to develop coronary disease.

A clear association with risk and blood pressure exists. Interestingly enough, the correlation with systolic pressure was better than with diastolic pressure or both pressures taken together, contrary to popular belief (19).

For years it has been implied that obesity is associated with the risk of developing coronary heart disease. Autopsy studies have not supported this view, and most pathologists would agree with this (20). A certain confusion arises here because weight and fatness cannot be equated. Sometimes an increased weight can be due to fluid retention and not solely to fat. A long-term follow-up of university students showed that the death rate from coronary heart disease was higher in those who had been relatively overweight at college but that relationship disappeared when the groups were made comparable according to blood pressure levels (21). Higher blood pressure can be associated with increased fluid retention due to hyperaldosteronism, and this increases body weight. Most of the results of correlation of increased weight and heart disease, therefore, serve only to emphasise the preeminent role of hypertension as a factor in the disease and one that must be tackled early and vigorously if prevention of coronary heart disease is to be a realistic proposition.

The role of diet and hyperlipidemia is not in doubt. Other dietary factors have been proposed but are not supportable as serious contenders in the aetiology of atherosclerosis. Yudkin's hypothesis that dietary sucrose is a factor cannot be supported on epidemiological, clinical, or experimental grounds (22). Likewise, the notion that large doses of vitamin E (and tocopherol) are of value in prevention remains unsupported (23). From time to time, various things are proposed as panaceas, such as vitamin C and so on, based on experimental work in animals. Clearly they need careful assessment, but to date nothing concrete has emerged from the plethora of proposals.

So far as the relationship of coronary heart disease to soft-water consumption is concerned, the evidence is not clear either way. Many elements exist in soft water, often in trace amounts, and their exact analysis is by no means easy to achieve. There is some evidence of a relationship between soft-water drinking and hypertension; elements such as cadmium in the water may play a part in this regard (24).

This review of risk factors in coronary heart disease has tended to assume that the disease is entirely of environmental origin. The widespread occurrence of fatty streaks in the vessels of young people of all races, however, might imply that man, as a genus, is genetically susceptible to atherosclerosis at least in its early fatty streak stage. Clearly, occasional examples of familial hyperlipidaemias provide evidence of genetic factors as perhaps does a tendency of men with blood group A to have higher blood cholesterol levels than those with blood group O (25). Again, genetic factors may be involved in hypertensive vascular disease.

So far as human races are concerned, there are few examples of genetic as opposed to environmental predisposition or lack of it to coronary heart disease. Often quoted are the Masai and Samburu tribes who live almost entirely on cow's milk, blood, and meat. Despite their high intake of saturated fats, they have low serum cholesterol levels. The explanation, so far as the Masai are concerned, seems to lie in a most effective feedback mechanism that suppresses the endogenous synthesis of cholesterol when the exogenous supply is high (26).

Despite all this, Keys concludes, "In general, though heredity may be a factor, it is not dominant enough to make people prisoners of their genes. In other words, there is every reason to urge an attack on relevant environmental factors in an effort to control coronary heart disease" (4). At the conclusion of the next chapter, after examining the experimental and other evidence, we shall endeavour to propose the form that such an attack might take.

References

1. Strong, J. P. and McGill, H. C., Jr.: The paediatric aspect of atherosclerosis. *J Atheroscler Res*, 9:251, 1969.

2. McGill, H. C., Jr.: Fatty streaks in the coronary arteries and aorta. *Lab Invest, 18:*100, 1968.
3. Holman, R. L.: Atherosclerosis — A paediatric nutrition problem? *Am J Clin Nutr, 9:*565, 1961.
4. Keys, A.: Coronary heart disease — The global picture. *Atherosclerosis, 22:*149, 1975.
5. Keys, A., Kimura, N., Kusukawa, A., Bronte-Stewart, B., Larsen, N. P., and Keys, M. H.: Lessons from serum cholesterol studies in Japan, Hawaii, and Los Angeles. *Ann Intern Med, 48:*83, 1958.
6. Toor, M., Katchalsky, A., Agmon, J., and Allalouf, D.: Atherosclerosis and related factors to immigrants in Israel. *Circulation, 22:*265, 1960.
7. Ehrström, M. C.: Medical studies in North Greenland 1948-49 Part 6. *Acta Med Scand, 140:*416, 1951.
8. Morris, J. N., Heady, J. A., Raffle, P. A. B., Roberts, C. G., and Parks, J. N.: Coronary heart disease and physical activity of work. *Lancet, 2:*1053, 1111, 1953.
9. Weiss, H. S., Brown, F. D., Griminger, P., and Fisher, H.: Physical activity and atherosclerosis in the adult chicken. *J Atheroscler Res, 6:*407, 1966.
10. Link, R. P., Pedersoli, W. M., and Safanie, A. H.: Effect of exercise on development of atherosclerosis in swine. *Atherosclerosis, 15:*107, 1972.
11. Robertson, H. K.: Heart disease in life-long cyclists. *Br Med J, 2:*1635, 1977.
12. Hinkle, L. E., Jr., Whitney, L. H., and Lehman, E. W.: Occupation, education and coronary heart disease. *Science, 161:*238, 1968.
13. Friedman, M. and Rosenman, R. H.: Type A behaviour pattern — Its association with coronary heart disease. *Ann Clin Res, 3:*300, 1971.
14. Keith, R. A., Lown, B., and Stare, F. J.: Coronary heart disease and behaviour patterns — An examination of method. *Psychosom Med, 27:*424, 1965.
15. Henry, J. P., Ely, D. L., Stephens, P. M., Ratcliffe, H. L., and Santisteban, G. A.: The role of psychological factors in the development of arteriosclerosis in C.B.A. mice. *Atherosclerosis, 14:*203, 1971.
16. Keys, A., Taylor, H. L., Blackburn, H., Brozek, J., and Anderson, J. T.: Mortality and coronary heart disease among men studied for twenty-three years. *Arch Intern Med, 128:*20, 1971.
17. Inter-Society Commission for Heart Disease Resources: Report on primary prevention of atherosclerotic disease. *Circulation, 42:*A55, 1970.
18. Keys, A., Aravanis, C., Blackburn, H., Van Buchem, F. S. P., Buzina, R., Djordjevic, B. S., Fidzana, F., Karvonen, M. J., Menotti, A., Puddu, V., and Taylor, H. L.: Coronary heart disease — Overweight and obesity as risk factors. *Ann Intern Med, 77:*15, 1972.
19. Kannel, W. B., Gordon, T., and Schwartz, M. J.: Systolic versus diastolic pressure and risk of coronary heart disease — The Framingham Study.

*Am J Cardiol, 27:*335, 1971.
20. Spain, D. M., Nathan, D. J., and Gellis, M.: Weight, body type and prevalance of atherosclerotic heart disease in males. *Am J Med Sci, 245:*63, 1963.
21. Paffenbarger, R. S., Jr., Notkin, J., Krueger, D. E., Wolf, P. A., Thorne, M. C., Lebaner, E. J., and Williams, J. L.: Chronic disease in former college students Part 2. *Am J Public Health, 56:*962, 1966.
22. Stamler, J., Berkson, D. M., Lindberg, H. A.: Risk factors — Their role in the aetiology and pathogenesis of the atherosclerotic diseases. In Wissler, R. W. and Geer, J. C. (Eds.): *The Pathogenesis of Atherosclerosis.* Baltimore, Williams and Wilkins, 1972, p. 41.
23. Hodges, R. E.: Vitamin E and coronary heart disease. *J Am Diet Assoc, 63:*538, 1973.
24. Perry, H. M.: Hypertension and the geochemical environment. In Hopps, H. C. and Cannon, H. L. (Eds.): Geochemical environment in relation to health and disease. *Ann NY Acad Sci, 199:*202, 1972.
25. Oliver, M. F., Geizerova, H., Cumming, R. A., and Heady, J. A.: Serum-cholesterol and A.B.O. and rhesus blood groups. *Lancet, 2:*605, 1969.
26. Biss, K., Ho, J. K., Mikkelsen, B., Lewis, L. A., and Taylor, C. B.: Some unique biological characteristics of the Masai of East Africa. *N Engl J Med, 284:*694, 1971.

CHAPTER 4

ATTEMPTS TO PREVENT AND CAUSE REGRESSION OF ATHEROSCLEROSIS

Introduction

THE production of atherosclerosis by various means, in experimental animals, has occupied many years of research in this century. As a result, a great deal of information has accumulated about the possible ways in which risk factors might operate directly or indirectly in promoting coronary heart disease. The purpose of this chapter is to review briefly the modes of action and then to consider, in detail, the various experiments in animals and in man that have been made in an attempt to reverse the atherosclerotic process.

A major difficulty in experimental animals, and even more so in man, is that of obtaining precise estimates of the degrees and extent of atherosclerotic disease in arteries. Without such information it is not easy to quantitate regression. In recent times, many methods of the mensuration of atherosclerotic disease have been devised for use both in excised arteries and latterly *in vivo*. These methods will be separately reviewed in the final chapter.

The principal provoking factors can be summarised briefly as in Table I (1).

TABLE I

ATHEROSCLEROSIS

PROVOKING FACTORS

Hyperlipidemia
Hypertension
Hypoxia
Hormones
Hypersensitivity
Hypercoagulability

36

Hyperlipidemia, which involves not only cholesterol and its esters but also triglycerides, free fatty acids, and lipoproteins, may act quite crudely by making more lipid available in plasma for deposition in the previously injured vessel wall. However, it is possible that hypercholesterolemia operates at an earlier stage, causing direct endothelial injury and facilitating the entry of plasma macromolecules into the intima. Hypertension can also be envisaged as having merely a crude stretching effect upon the vessel, thus enhancing permeability of the endothelial sheet to plasma constituents. We have already seen, however, that endothelial cells are damaged in hypertension and that the endothelial cell turnover is increased in this circumstance. In those cases of hypertension where renin levels are elevated, there is likely to be an increased level of angiotensin II. There is clear evidence that this peptide causes endothelial cells to separate (2).

The role of hypoxia is a fairly recent notion, which we have already mentioned briefly among the factors that might provoke coronary heart disease. It will be discussed fully in this section because much of the evidence from experimental studies, at least, needs critical re-evaluation. Smokers have a raised level of carboxyhaemoglobin in their blood, and experimental work suggests that this might cause increased endothelial permeability (3). Tobacco smoke also has a toxic effect on smooth muscle cells in tissue culture; we shall say more of this later.

In some way, female hormones seem to have a protective role in atherogenesis, though in excess they may promote thrombosis, particularly in the venous circulation. Precisely how the premenopausal female is relatively protected against coronary heart disease is not clear, but recent evidence has emerged implicating high-density lipoproteins in this role (4). The mode of action of the high-density lipoproteins seems to be to facilitate the transport of cholesterol to the liver for catabolism, thus reducing the plasma level. Oestrogens have a more subtle effect on smooth muscle cells, at least in tissue culture, in that they reduce the proliferation induced by lipoproteins (5). It could be envisaged that the development of the atherosclerotic lesion might be inhibited in this way.

The possible parts played by immunological injury in atherogenesis are still debatable. There is no doubt that immune complexes can damage small blood vessels; whether they injure the larger arteries to produce atherosclerosis is problematical. The evidence is reviewed by Davies (5), who makes the points that immune complexes are toxic to endothelial cells and also promote platelet aggregation and subsequent blood coagulation. In rabbits it is possible to cause atherosclerosis by immunological injury (6).

Finally, the role of platelets in atherogenesis has already been discussed, and the possible role of a high molecular weight, heat-stable, thrombin-activated platelet factor needs to be kept in mind.

Experiments with Risk Factors in Animals — Lipids

Many of the experimental studies on regression of atherosclerosis have involved feeding atherogenic diets, often containing added cholesterol, for varying times and then stopping the atherogenic stimulus and waiting to see if the disease regresses. Apart from the problem of accurate measurement of degrees of the disease, there is also that of choosing a suitable experimental animal from which results can be reasonably extrapolated to an understanding of human atherogenesis.

Some of the early work was done by Horlick and Katz (7). They fed a large group of chicks on a mash supplemented with 2 percent cholesterol and 20 percent cottonseed oil for ten weeks. A sample was then killed and the degree of atheroma was determined. A second group continued on the atherogenic diet for another fourteen weeks. Two other groups were kept on regular mash and defatted mash, respectively, for the next fourteen weeks. Cessation of cholesterol feeding led to a rapid fall in plasma cholesterol levels to normal. In the ensuing weeks some lesions disappeared; in others fibrous tissue and calcification remained. Since then, similar results in many animals have been described. Anitschow showed a spontaneous regression of atherosclerosis in rabbits (8). A common feature of all these experiments was a rapid fall of serum cholesterol when the atherogenic diet was withdrawn. By contrast, lesions disappeared rather slowly; in some animals they persisted and in others the disease worsened.

In the rabbit, which has long been used as an experimental subject, there was a tendency for the induced lesions to persist unchanged or even to progress when the animals were returned to a normal diet. In 1962, Schuler and Albrecht demonstrated the remarkable susceptibility of the rabbit to an atherogenic stimulus. Cholesterol was fed for as short a period of ten days, yet this triggered irreversible atheromatous disease in the rabbit. The degree of atheroma in the rabbit aorta was concluded to be independent of the level of plasma cholesterol (9). Many workers agree, however, that early, lipid-rich lesions in the rabbit may regress. Studies by scanning and transmission electron microscopy have shown that atherosclerotic lesions in rabbits can regress after withdrawal from a short-term atherogenic diet. Initially, the core of the plaques consisted of lipid-laden cells devoid of endothelial covering, but the lipid slowly disappeared and the endothelial covering was re-established (10). Similar reversibility has been reported by others (11). As long as the endothelial layer is incomplete over the lesion, myointimal cellular proliferation continues. Once the surface is re-established, development of the lesion stops (12).

It was suggested by Constantinides et al. (13) that, once fibrosis had developed within the rabbit lesion regression did not occur; the lesions that appeared within two months of the start of the atherogenic diet persisted for two years after a return to a normal diet. Furthermore, the lesions were larger than those found in animals killed after two months on the diet. Adams fed pulse-labelled tritium cholesterol to rabbits for twelve weeks; this was taken up into the aortic wall where it remained for a year after stopping the diet. Free cholesterol rose in proportion to the level of cholesterol ester, and histological and histochemical methods failed to demonstrate resorption of cholesterol (14). Adams concluded that the metabolic activities of the mature atherosclerotic lesion, in the rabbit, seemed exceedingly limited in contrast with the actively metabolic, rapidly exchangeable pool of cholesterol in liver and plasma. The rabbit is clearly ill equipped to deal with hyperchplesterolemia, being a herbivore. However, the liver of the animal can handle it efficiently, so it may be that the metabolically relatively inert vessel wall accounts for the sluggish turnover of vascular lipids.

Previous work in the rat had shown a persistence of vascular lipidosis after the atherogenic stimulus had been withdrawn, which led the authors to conclude that lipid content of the vessel wall, once established, is independent of the stimulus that produced it (15). In the rat, also, the liver pool of cholesterol reduced rapidly after withdrawing the atherogenic stimulus, so that similar conclusions might be reached to those gained from the rabbit experiments.

Considering these experiments alone, the outlook for possible regression of atherosclerosis seemed gloomy, certainly so far as the lipid and collagen contents of the lesions were concerned. Subsequent work in other animals, however, presented a more optimistic picture, and the important observation that a combined assault on the problem would yield better results has changed the position. This latter work by Wissler and his colleagues (16) has shown that although dietary restriction alone, in the rabbit, has little effect on atherosclerosis reversal, much better results are obtained if the limitation of diet is coupled with hyperoxia and cholestyramine or oestrogen or both.

Work in nonhuman primates has yielded results that suggest that regression and prevention of atherosclerosis are real possibilities. Initially, work done by Maruffo and Portman with the squirrel monkey proved disappointing (17). They fed an atherogenic diet for three months and then followed this with a control diet for the next three to five months. These animals showed lesions that did not progress as compared to monkeys kept on the atherogenic regime. However, the lesions did not regress to produce a state found in the control animals. It could be argued that enough time had not been allowed for regression to occur.

Much more encouraging was the work of Armstrong et al. The basic experiments consisted of feeding a control diet for six weeks followed by an atherogenic one for seventeen months; the animals were then given regression diets for as long as forty months (18). The regression diets were either rich in linoleate or of a low-fat type. Stenosing atheromatous lesions developed when the atherogenic diet was given. The regression diets of either kind resulted in small fibrotic lesions, which had scanty stainable lipid in them. The increase in size of the lumen of these vessels was not merely due to vascular dilatation because measurement of the intimal area revealed that there was a three-fold reduction as compared to the arteries of the monkeys given the atherogenic diet and no regression diet. Similar work was done by Eggen et al. (19), who confirmed that lipid could be induced to leave atheromatous lesions in the aorta and in other vessels. This was done by feeding a cholesterol-enriched diet for twelve weeks and sequentially examining the groups of animals for up to sixty-four weeks. In this study, there was a dramatic change in the appearance of the lesions after the regression diet. All foam cells in the lesions had gone by thirty-two and sixty-four weeks; in addition, most of the smooth muscle cells had lost their lipid, and extracellular lipid in the intima was also reduced. Medial lipid was not removed, and a longer period on the regression diet might have been needed to achieve this. Histological evaluation also seemed to show that a reduction of lipid in the regressing lesions was accompanied by an increase of intimal collagen. However, in a subsequent study, Armstrong and Megan (20), using *Macaca fascicularis*, concluded that collagen was lost from aortic lesions in regression but the collagen increased in lesions of the coronary arteries.

More detailed chemical studies of the lipids in lesions induced in rhesus monkeys have been made by Kokatnur et al. (21). The diet was fed for twelve weeks and then changed to a low-cholesterol, low-fat content. The animals were studied for up to sixty-four weeks thereafter. The early change was an alteration of distribution between intimal cells and intercellular material; this happened in sixteen weeks. Then followed a net loss of intimal lipid. This redistribution between cells and intercellular substance, on regression, may provide a notion of the mechanisms of lipid removal. Interestingly, the esters of saturated and monounsaturated fatty acids were preferentially expelled from the vessel wall. Less of the polyunsaturated esters came out, and free cholesterol was likewise relatively resistant to egress.

The general impression that can, at present, be gained from the study of nonhuman primates is that dietary-induced atherosclerosis is reversible and that the mechanisms involved include loss of lipid from cells, which then enters the intercellular space and slowly equilibrates with that in plasma. Most people find that intimal lipids emerge from inner vessel walls more easily than those from the media. This may simply be a matter of mechanical diffusion or it may reflect different metabolic activities in various parts of the artery wall.

Electron microscopic studies by Tucker et al. (22) and Strong, Eggen, and Stary (23) provide morphological support for the mechanism of lipid loss from the intima on regression. Early atherosclerotic lesions show abundant foam cells, which are probably monocytes, and smooth muscle cells containing droplets of lipid. These appearances were produced in as little as eight weeks, and regressive changes appeared about sixteen weeks after the atherogenic diet had been withdrawn. These consisted of progressive breakdown of the monocytes, which spilled lipid into the extracellular space, and loss of lipid from the muscle cells. Strong et al. (23) examined a range of vessels in their experiments on regression and showed that aortic lesions regressed less easily than those in other arteries. Uptake of tritiated thymidine by intimal cells, which was increased in the atherosclerotic lesions, was reduced when the atherogenic stimulus, hypercholesterolemia in this case, was removed.

It now seems likely that fibrous tissue and necrotic atheromatous debris can also be removed from lesions during regression. Experiments by Daoud et al. (24) in the pig illustrate this point. They produced advanced, complicated atheroma in pigs by a combination of a high-cholesterol, high-fat diet following mechanical injury to the aortic intima with a balloon catheter. When the high-cholesterol diet was removed and the animals were given swine mash for fourteen months, there was a significant reduction in size of the lesions with the reformation of a smooth intimal surface.

All of the experiments that have been discussed so far involve groups of animals killed at various times in the experiment. From these results, a sequence of regression is inferred. Attempts to study regressive changes in the same artery in life are few. De Palma et al. produced atheroma in the mesenteric arteries of dogs by feeding cholesterol and ablating the thyroid (25). They then stopped the atherogenic diet and observed sequential regressive changes in the arteries of each animal by repeated laparotomy and aortotomy. It is remarkable that regression occurred at all because every insult to an artery is, of itself, a potential atherogenic stimulus. However, drug therapy or internal biliary diversion was needed, as well as withdrawal from the diet, to achieve the result.

The majority of dietary experiments involve feeding fats of one sort or another combined with cholesterol supplements and then withdrawing the stimulus to see if regression occurs. Another interesting dietary approach is to study an animal such as the White Carneau pigeon, which develops severe aortic and coronary atherosclerosis closely resembling the human disease (26). These studies were based on previous work in the rat by McCance and Widdowson (27), who showed that the size and weight of adult rats were determined by the plane of nutrition before they were weaned. Underfed animals developed into small but normal adults. A similar phenomenon was shown to occur in the White Carneau pigeon and, more important, there was a reduction in the degree of atherosclerosis in these animals (28). This occurred despite the fact that the underfed animals showed a great spurt of growth so that the previously deprived bird is the same weight as its control adult. So far as man is concerned, these experiments might support the hypothesis that the rising incidence of atherosclerotic disease in the Western World is the result of exuberant infant nutrition.

The notion that deficiency of essential fatty acids, such as linoleic, in the diet can provide an atherogenic stimulus does not currently command much interest. Diets deficient in essential fatty acids have been shown to produce atherosclerotic lesions in rabbits (29), pigs (30), and rats. Morin et al. (31) were able to produce lipid-containing lesions in rat coronary arteries by feeding a diet containing 20 percent hydrogenated coconut oil. Lipid deposition was also increased in the livers of these animals. This suggested that cholesterol transport was defective in the tissues of animals deficient in essential fatty acids. The lesions could be induced to regress if the rats were subsequently fed essential fatty acids in the form of cottonseed oil.

This discussion will now consider other dietary substances such as carbohydrate and protein. The atherogenic role of dietary carbohydrate has little support; the only possible effect is the production of obesity and of hypertriglyceridaemia, neither of which are clearly associated with coronary heart disease. Few animal experiments have been done. However, it is reported that obesity can be produced in baboons by feeding sucrose over the period of a year but that this was not associated with enhanced atherosclerosis (32). From present studies it seems unlikely that any modification of the average dietary intake of carbohydrate will have any effect on atherogenesis.

Studies on protein content of the diet are rather more complex. Previous work has shown that protein-deficient diets tend to aggravate experimentally induced atherosclerosis in roosters and hens fed cholesterol (33). It has been shown also that excessively high protein levels in the diet inhibit diet-induced hypercholesterolemia and atherosclerosis (34). Pick et al. (35) undertook a study of the effects of high and low dietary protein on the regression of dietary-induced atherosclerosis in cockerels. They found that regression of lesions was impaired when dietary protein was low (7-10%). Others have found that a meat-enriched diet will impede the development of atherosclerosis in rabbits fed cholesterol, and the addition of casein or methionine to the diets will prevent these changes (36). Polcák et al. (37) fed a standard diet to rabbits together with 20 g meat and added cholesterol. The serum and tissue levels of cholesterol were lower in those with meat added, and atherosclerotic changes in the aortas were also less in these animals.

Some interesting results have come from a study of the effects of blackgram in the diet. It is of leguminous origin and contains about 25 percent protein, 65 percent carbohydrate, and 2.5 percent fat. It has a remarkable hypocholesterolemic effect and forms an important part of the staple diet in India. Fed to rats it has a profound hypocholesterolaemic effect, which was thought to be due to the globulin fraction of the material (38). Similar effects were found in rats given the globulin fraction from related pulses (redgram and horsegram) (39). Blackgram also contained an insoluble carbohydrate fraction which, like the globulin component, had a lipid-lowering effect, but the insoluble carbohydrate fractions from redgram and horsegram had no such effect.

The effects of dietary proteins in relation to atherogenesis need more investigation. It seems likely that a proper proportion of fat and protein is needed to preserve healthy arteries. Which of the proteins has an optimal effect, if any, remains debatable.

From time to time all sorts of food constituents and additives have been suggested to have a hypocholesterolaemic and anti-atherogenic effect. In 1934, the artichoke was endowed with powers to lower serum cholesterol (41), and similar properties were ascribed to the eggplant (42) and avocado pear (43). Cookson et al. (44) recount the beneficial effects of feeding hop blossom and alfalfa in the diet. Alfalfa prevented the hypercholesterolaemia and atherosclerosis produced in control rabbits by cholesterol feeding. The control levels of cholesterol were in excess of 1000 mgm/100 ml, whereas in animals fed alfalfa and a similar amount of cholesterol, the levels were normal. These workers claim that alfalfa produced its effect by inhibiting cholesterol absorbtion from the gut. Currently, claims are made for a similar action of other forms of dietary roughage. Soya bean also has a hypocholesterolaemic effect, but the mode of action has not been elucidated (45). The list of various dietary panaceas reads somewhat like a quotation from Shakespeare's *Macbeth* or from the prodigious works of Paracelsus. Nevertheless, there may arise another William Withering to dissect out from the vast mixture a potent anti-atherosclerotic agent.

Experiments with Risk Factors in Animals — Hypertension

There is no question that the production of experimental hypertension promotes the development of atherosclerosis though relatively few animal experiments are available (40). Even fewer experiments are recorded showing the effects of reversing induced hypertension on atherogenesis. Much more needs to be done because, as we shall see, hypotensive drugs in man are effective in preventing stroke but seem to have little action in the occurrence of coronary heart disease. However, these are early days in the use of hypotensives, and it may well be that the apparent lack of an anti-atherogenic effect of efficient control of hypertension may be because the treatment begins late in life when symptoms have developed and the disease is well established.

Experiments with Risk Factors in Animals — Hypoxia

A discussion of the role of cigarette smoking in atherogenesis has been left to this section of the book because the epidemiological and experimental aspects are intricately interwoven. It is a sound general pathological principle that hypoxia will damage cells and lead to fatty accumulation within them (46). The question is whether an elevated level of blood carboxyhaemoglobin or other factors from cigarettes can damage the arterial wall. This question has, up to the present time, proved extraordinarily difficult to answer.

Several epidemiological studies support the association of atherosclerosis and cigarette smoking in man (47). Problems arise in such studies from an inability to randomise the subjects who are being studied and from the difficulty of disassociating other factors connected with cigarette smoking that might have atherogenic potency. Strong et al. (48) attempted to make the analysis more precise by looking at the aortas and coronary arteries of 747 men aged 20 to 64 who had been subjected to autopsy. Smoking histories of the dead men were obtained, in a suitably controlled way, from their relatives. It was found that atherosclerotic involvement of the aorta and coronary arteries was greatest in heavy smokers and least in nonsmokers and that occupational physical activity and educational standards seemed to have no relationship. Various problems arise in the interpretation of their results. Some of the numbers of cases in the subgroups in the study were rather small, and the smokers and nonsmokers were self-related and not randomised. Other factors such as stress, temperament, diet, and other life habits may also cause differences in atherosclerosis. The other problem, which occurs with any autopsy study, is that the sample is not necessarily a reflection of the living population or for that matter of the deceased population in the particular area under study. This can be a potent distorting factor in some parts of the world where local customs in autopsy practice are sharply confined to one stratum of the populace. The paper is concluded with the unanswerable question whether the findings in the dead would be greatly different from a random sample of the living. A further extension of this study was reported in 1976 (49). The authors have examined 1,320 autopsies from men aged 25 to 64 and now conclude that "this type of study does not and cannot provide conclusive evidence of a causal relationship between cigarette smoking and atherosclerosis." They emphasise the need for further experimental studies in animals to determine this point.

A variety of vascular changes has been produced both by systemic hypoxia and by the inhalation of carbon monoxide. Most of the work has been done in the rabbit, and the changes have been both medial and intimal. The main difficulties in interpretation lie in quantitation of the degree of change and extrapolation of the results to an understanding of human disease. Garbarsch et al. (50, 51) describe the effects of systemic hypoxia in rabbits made severely hypoxic by the intermittent inhalation of nitrogen. They found an increased synthesis of medial acid-sulphated mucopolysaccharides, and the uptake of (^{35}S) sulphate is increased. They did not find any evidence of increased endothelial permeability to albumin in the experimental animals. They concluded that the medial change was partly due to hypoxia and partly to the effects of systemic hypertension induced by intense hypoxia. In a subsequent paper (52), the same authors categorise the different sorts of glycosaminoglycans that arise following hypoxia. Though they speak of producing arteriosclerosis, they do not recount any intimal changes save an increase in intimal area.

A number of papers from the Danish School of Workers describe intimal changes in rabbit arteries following exposure to carbon monoxide. This work was done by scanning and transmission light microscopy. Previous studies using light microscopy had shown vascular changes following acute fatal carbon monoxide poisoning in man. The changes were said to be thickening of the vessel wall, loosening of vascular membranes, and swelling of capillary endothelium (53). In chronic moderate exposure, the changes were essentially those of oedema of the vessel wall (54). In a more recent study (55), the same authors reported electron microscope findings of intimal oedema, subendothelial blisters, and deformation of the folding structure of the endothelial surface. They also described plaques composed of degenerate, fragmented, calcified elastic fibres, collagen, and amorphous debris. Some of these changes are artefactual since fixation of the vessels was not made at a standard pressure. However, others have shown endothelial damage following hypoxia (56) with thrombocytes adherent to the damaged areas.

If rabbits are fed a diet containing 2 percent cholesterol and also exposed to intermittent carbon monoxide so that the blood carboxyhaemoglobin rises to 20 percent on each exposure, no significant changes in plasma or aortic lipids are found. However, the extent of coronary atherosclerosis was greatest in the group exposed to the gas. This experiment was done by Davies et al. (57) in an attempt to repeat a similar one (58) by Astrup. They were unable to repeat the experiment, which purported to describe an increase in cholesterol content of the aorta following intermittent exposure to carbon monoxide. These findings are similar to those described by Thomsen (59) in the monkey *(Macaca irus)*. Furthermore, the enhancing effect of carbon monoxide on coronary atherosclerosis is not maintained; thus, the results of the acute rabbit experiment described by Davies et al. (57) may be but a temporary acute response.

It is also important to get these experiments into the proper perspective and not to assume that the effects produced by carbon monoxide are necessarily the same as those produced by tobacco smoke. Turner and Topping (60), for example, have shown in the squirrel monkey that the effects on lipid metabolism of CO alone and of tobacco smoke are quite different even though the degree of exposure may be the same.

Studies in the White Carneau pigeon, which develops spontaneous atheroma without provocation, raise problems similar to those already discussed. The birds were exposed to carbon monoxide intermittently, some were normocholesterolemic, others had raised cholesterol levels induced by adding 1 percent cholesterol to the diet. It was found that carbon monoxide had no enhancing effect on the normocholesterolemic animals whereas those with raised cholesterol levels showed an increased degree of coronary atheroma after fifty-two weeks of exposure. However, at the end of eighty-four weeks exposure no such enhancement was found (61).

It was interesting that, after fifty-two weeks, the mean cholesterol of some of the birds declined, which presumably accounted for the results for coronary atheroma at eighty-four weeks. This suggests that compensatory mechanisms come into action to reverse the effects of carbon monoxide despite continued administration. Further evidence of adaptation of arterial tissue to hypoxia is reflected by the changes of lactate dehydrogenase activity in the hypoxic vessel wall. In hypoxia the total level of the enzyme increased, and the appropriate isoenzyme composition was shifted towards a pattern with a higher percentage of M subunits (62).

There is a considerable debate about the effects of carbon monoxide on vessel wall dynamics. The experiments of Sarma et al. (63) studied the perfusion of human coronary arteries after death with blood containing varied concentrations of carbon monoxide. Lipid synthesis was followed by perfusion of (^{14}C) acetate and (^{3}H) cholesterol. They were unable to find any effect of carbon monoxide on lipid synthesis. However, the uptake of cholesterol was increased, suggesting that the permeability of endothelial membranes was increased. Using an entirely different technique, Howard and Bonnett showed that slices of atherosclerotic lesions of rabbit aorta took up lipid precursors more avidly than the normal and that lipogenesis was further enhanced if the cultures were made hypoxic (64). Different techniques in different animals provide different results; here lies one of the major problems for the interpretation of findings in terms of human disease.

Another aspect of smoking that has not yet been considered is the effect upon clotting mechanisms. Much has been written on this subject, and the findings are still confused. Recent experiments by Moschos et al. (65) show enhancement of fibrinogen turnover and a fall in platelet count in beagle hounds subjected chronically to tobacco smoke. No observations were reported of fibrinolytic changes so that the significance of these changes in terms of deposition of coagulation products on the vascular intima remains obscure.

When hypoxia is combined with hypertension, the athero-genic effect is augmented. Frith et al. (66) studied the effects of hypoxemia and hypertension in miniature swine. The hypox-emic animals had normal plasma lipid levels and did not de-velop systemic hypertension. However, they developed pulmonary hypertension. Enzyme studies of both aorta and pulmonary artery showed increased nucleotide pyrophospha-tase and lactate dehydrogenase activity. Smooth muscle cells in the mid media of both vessels showed degenerative changes by electron microscopy. Whereas the aorta showed no alterations to light microscopy, the pulmonary artery showed thickening of all three layers and, by contrast with the aorta, showed in-creased cholesterol and free fatty acid in the intima-media.

In conclusion, the role of smoking in atherogenesis is still unclear. If any component of tobacco is responsible it is not clear which it is, and more animal experiments are needed.

A number of attempts to reverse or inhibit atherogenesis by hyperoxia have been made recently. Early work by Altschul and Herman on rabbits made hypercholesterolemic on a 0.3 g cho-lesterol feed per day showed that daily inhalation of oxygen for three hours reduced the level of their serum cholesterol (67). Furthermore, there had been an inhibition of atheroma devel-opment in some of the hyperoxic animals. Kjeldsen et al. (68) fed rabbits cholesterol, exposed them to degrees of hyperoxia, and then examined lipids and the state of atheroma in the aorta. Serum and aortic lipids were lower in the hyperoxic group and they had less atherosclerosis. The mode of action of hyperoxia is debatable. The rabbit aorta is poorly nourished by vasa vasorum, and any degree of intimal thickening will impair diffusion of nutrients from the lumen. Hyperoxia may act merely to improve diffusion through the wall. However, hyper-cholesterolemia causes other changes that may lead to impaired oxygenation of the vessel wall: increased oxygen consumption in the aorta, reduced oxygen saturation of the blood, and a slower diffusion of oxygen in the blood (68).

We have already considered the problems of reversibility of cholesterol-induced atherosclerosis in rabbits. Sometimes withdrawal of the diet leads to regression; at other times it does not (69). When diet withdrawal is coupled with hyperoxia and cholestyramine or oestrogen, successful regression can be achieved (70). It has become increasingly clear throughout this discussion that any success that might be achieved in man is more likely if a combined rather than a single measure is used. Similarly, De Palma et al., who showed regression of lesions in dogs (25), were unable to achieve the result merely by withdrawing the diet; they needed internal biliary diversion and drugs as well (71).

Experiments with Risk Factors in Animals — Hormones

The actions of most hormones as means of causing or preventing atherosclerosis have been considered from time to time. Because of the obvious relative immunity of the premenopausal human female to coronary heart disease, it is not surprising that oestrogens have received most of the attention. However, though there is evidence of the beneficial effect of oestrogen in animals (72), clinical results in man are still controversial (73).

We shall consider other hormones briefly and return to study the effects of oestrogens. Thyroid hormones have a clear relationship to blood lipid levels. Hypothyroid states achieved by thyroidectomy, dosage with ^{131}I or thiouracil, have been used in dogs and rats to produce hyperlipidemia and atherosclerosis (74). Thyroid hormone given to chicks on an atherogenic diet suppresses hypercholesterolemia and in some experiments decreases atherogenesis as well; this discrepancy may be due to the direct damaging effect of the thyroid hormone on the vessel wall, which may itself lead to atherosclerosis (75).

Adrenal cortical hormones also have an effect. The glucocorticoids enhance hypercholesterolemia but curiously enough do not have an atherogenic effect. This phenomenon has been demonstrated in many experimental animals (76). Mineralcorticoids produce hypertension when given to chicks and by this means intensify atherosclerosis. If, however, sufficient fluid retention is not achieved to produce hypertension, then there is no effect on atherogenesis.

The role of pancreatic hormones is complex and unclear at present. Statistically, there is an increased risk of coronary heart disease in patients with diabetes mellitus, and there is a factor in the serum from diabetics, which is neither insulin nor glucose, that stimulates the growth of smooth muscle cells in culture. This might be regarded as an atherogenic factor.

Abnormalities of carbohydrate and lipid metabolism such as reduced glucose tolerance, hyperlipoproteinemia and hypertriglyceridemia are found in diabetics, and any of these have, from time to time, been linked with atherosclerotic disease. Recent studies of patients with premature vascular disease have also shown an exaggerated insulin response to oral glucose (78, 79, 80). Insulin stimulates lipogenesis in the arterial wall, and this is increased in hyperinsulinism (81). Thus, it has been proposed that the primary abnormality in atherosclerosis is an exaggerated insulin response to dietary carbohydrate and that the vascular disease and metabolic disorders follow this (82).

The role of insulin is clearly complex: too much or too little of it seems to be related to atherogenesis. Early experiments with pancreatectomised chicks produced interesting but equally complex results. Removal of the pancreas in a chick is readily done, yet the animals show no abnormality of lipids or carbohydrate metabolism. Furthermore, they will behave in the same way as normal animals when given 0.25 percent cholesterol in the diet. Both groups get hypercholesterolemia and atherosclerosis to the same degree. However, when 2 percent cholesterol and 5 percent cottonseed oil are added to the diet, the pancreatectomised animals show enhanced hypercholesterolemia and atherosclerosis of the aorta and of the coronary arteries (83). Interesting results were also obtained when insulin was given to normal chicks on an atherogenic diet. It did not influence the development of atherosclerotic lesions, but it did hinder regression of the lesions when the animals were taken off the atherogenic regime. A number of factors operate on atherogenic mechanisms in patients with diabetes mellitus, and there is little prophylactic information to be gained from the experiments that we have discussed save the need to maintain normal blood lipid levels in those subjects.

Of all the hormones that have been examined, oestrogens have the most profound effect on experimental atherosclerosis in the chick. When cholesterol and oestrogen are given simultaneously, the chicks develop athcrosclerosis of the aorta to the same degree as controls given cholesterol alone. However, those given the combined regime showed inhibition of the development of coronary atheroma (84). Furthermore, the administration of oestrogen to those animals that had developed coronary disease on the cholesterol supplement alone caused the lesions to regress even though cholesterol feeding was maintained (85). This is a unique phenomenon in the field of atherosclerosis research and indicates the remarkable potency of oestrogen as an anti-atherogenic agent in coronary arteries. Oestrogens continue to exert their protective effect on coronary disease even when combined with testosterone, adrenal hormones, or pancreatectomy. The only regime that counteracts it is the induction of hypothyroidism by thiouracil. It seems that a euthyroid state is essential for the effective anti-atherosclerotic action of oestrogens (86). It also illustrates that the aorta and coronary arteries can behave discrepantly and that it is, therefore, not reasonable to talk of aortic atheroma if one is intent to study coronary artery disease.

The effect of oestrogen on plasma lipids in the cholesterol-fed birds was to maintain a normal cholesterol to phospholipid ration; without oestrogen the ratio was elevated. This may partly be because oestrogens have been shown to increase the incorporation of (^{32})P into phospholipids in man, cat, and rat but into no other lipid (87). Other metabolic effects of oestrogens have been noted in relation to atherogenesis. Some of them are curiously paradoxical. For example, the administration of the oestrogenic substance norethynodrel to rabbits will reduce the atherogenic effects of dietary cholesterol in that species, yet it increased the accumulation of acid mucopolysaccharides in the media, which some have regarded as a precursor of atherosclerosis (88). Some of the difficulties in understanding the effects of oestrogens stem from the failure to specify which particular oestrogen is being studied. Kroman et al. (89), for

example, found a relationship between blood lipids and oestrogens in men and women. Those with normal lipids had a
higher concentration of 17-β-oestradiol in the blood than oestrogen. Conversely, those persons with coronary artery disease
appeared to have a greater concentration of oestrone than 1-β-
oestradiol (89).

Equally confusing are the reports of the effects of various
oestrogens on the coagulation mechanisms in the blood. A
significant increase in serum oestrone and oestradiol was found
as a precursor of myocardial infarction in young men (90). In
addition, the potentially thrombogenic and hypertensive effects
of synthetic oestrogens are well documented (91).

It is difficult to put the results of experiments by Renaud (92)
into proper perspective against the backcloth of experimental
detail. He determined the susceptibility of rats to endotoxin-
initiated thrombosis. The animals were fed butter to make
them hyperlipidemic, and premarin, a conjugated oestrogen,
was added to the diet of some animals. At two dose levels the
drug reduced the serum cholesterol and triglyceride levels and
diminished the degree of atherosclerosis. In addition, the lower
dosage prolonged the coagulation time and prevented thrombosis. Here, then, is another important point when discussing
the effects of oestrogen, namely the need to specify the dosage
of the substance under test.

Experiments with Risk Factors in Animals — Hypersensitivity

The notion that atherosclerosis might be the result of a hypersensitivity reaction to various antigens is comparatively
new. Not much has been written about it and the amount of
experimental work is also scanty. Most of the evidence for the
hypothesis is indirect, the most significant being that from the
experiments of Levy (93) and Van Winkle and Levy (94).

Levy showed that a single injection of bovine serum albumen
produced endothelial cell proliferation in the rabbit aorta.
When the diet was enriched with 1 percent cholesterol, the
lesions consisted of both endothelial and foam cells. The lesions resembled those of early atherosclerosis and were found in

the aorta and coronary arteries. Out of these experiments came the proposal that repeated antigenic stimuli in man, over the years, might cause vascular damage by antigen-antibody complexes leading to lipid deposition. Howard et al. (95) confirmed the atherogenic potency of intermittent injections of bovine serum albumen in baboons that had been fed on a diet containing added cholesterol.

There is little doubt that antigen-antibody complexes have a variety of other potentially atherogenic effects on the vessel wall. They may activate endothelial cells and promote the deposition of fibrin and platelets (96). Antibody and complement may also have a direct cytotoxic effect on endothelial cells (97). Furthermore, antigen-antibody complexes will enhance blood coagulation and cause aggregation of platelets and immune adherence of erythrocytes (97). Finally, the complexes activate mast cells leading to the release of agents such as 5-hydroxytryptamine, which can induce increased endothelial permeability; the activation of complement components by complexes can produce a similar effect (98).

Some of the most convincing evidence for the role of immune mechanisms in the atherogenic process comes from the studies of arteries in transplanted organs. For example, homografts of thoracic aorta inserted into the abdominal aorta of hypercholesterolemic dogs develop atheroma that is no different in degree from that of the adjacent abdominal aorta. However, if a piece of abdominal aorta is inserted into the thoracic part, the degree of atheroma that appears in the donor segment is much greater than that in the adjacent host tissue (99). Other workers showed the development of extensive atheroma in fresh homografts and allografts of rabbit aorta (100, 101). We shall discuss human transplantation experiments later.

A novel idea is that the phasic nature of the atherogenic process might support the immunological concept of its origin. Gerö has written much along these lines and links the phasic nature of atherosclerosis to that of allergic lesions, emphasising the relation of myocardial infarction to allergic events. In addition, he points out that the early step in the atherosclerotic process is an intimal oedema that might be of allergic origin (102). The death rate from ischaemic heart disease rises in winter, and this is unrelated to fluctuations in triglyceride of cholesterol levels (103). However, milk antibodies do fluctuate in this way in patients with ischaemic heart disease, and Davis has postulated that allergy to milk protein might be an atherogenic factor (104).

No one has yet suggested that atherosclerosis might be prevented by immunosuppresive agents, nor has there been a proposal for the use of cytotoxic agents if the monoclonal hypothesis of atherosclerosis is sustained. The suggestion that atheroma might be regarded as a neoplastic process is perhaps a fitting end to this review (105).

Experiments with Drugs

A large variety of drugs has been used to prevent or reduce the degree of atherosclerosis. Their use has largely been dictated by a knowledge of the various risk factors that prevail in the disease and of the results of the various animal experiments that we have considered already. Unfortunately, most of the drugs that have been used have shown no useful effect, and when it is remembered that any drug therapy that is to be successful must start early in life, be inexpensive and free from side effects the prospect is not encouraging. Far more success is likely to result from the reduction of risk factors such as hypertension, hyperlipidemia, and smoking.

In this chapter we shall look at the various drugs grouped according to their mode of action. Perhaps the most popular and extensively used are those concerned with lowering lipid levels or changing the nature of the lipid in vessel walls and in plasma by the interpolation of different fatty acids.

First there is the group of methods designed to reduce the absorption of cholesterol from the gut. In 1959, Berger and colleagues (106) described the anion exchange resin cholestyramine, which binds bile acids in the gut. The clinical effects in man are controversial, but the substance has a potent effect in reversing atherosclerosis in animals that had previously been fed cholesterol and were later given a low-fat, low-cholesterol diet (70). Colestipol is another high molecular weight polymer with a high capacity for binding bile acids. It has an inhibitory effect on the development of hypercholesterolemia in cockerels that have been fed cholesterol and has a similar effect in dogs (107).

Another way of reducing the absorbtion of cholesterol is to bypass the ileum. This is a somewhat heroic measure but it is effective. Atherosclerosis can be prevented in the hypercholesterolemic rabbit if a partial ileal bypass is performed (108), and similar results have been obtained in the dog (109). There are many who would say that the only hope for people with familial hypercholesterolemia is to do an ileal bypass, and we shall return to this later. Meanwhile, it is important to realise that such an operation is by no means always successful. Attempts to affect cholesterol levels in White Carneau pigeons on a normal diet by means of ileal bypass have failed in experiments lasting as long as 18 months (110). However, the mode of action of ileal bypass is thought to be the prevention of bile acid absorption in that part of the gut. This is true for mammals, but it does appear that in the chick and egglaying hen the major site of bile acid absorbtion is the jejunum and not the ileum (111).

A number of experiments have been conducted working on the principle that lipids containing essential fatty acids are less histotoxic and are more easily removable from the tissues. In 1971, Howard et al. (95) were able to show that thrice weekly injections of polyunsaturated soya phosphatidyl choline reduced the severity of atherosclerosis in baboons given cholesterol and immunological arterial injury. It was concluded that a rise in cholesterol esterase activity in the arterial wall was the principal reason for this. In later experiments with baboons, Howard et al. studied another enzyme in the aorta. This was acyl-CoA cholesterol acyltransferase (ACAT), which was inhibited. They concluded that the anti-atherosclerotic effect of the polyunsaturated compound was due to the inhibition of ACAT production (112). Others using rats and pigs gave the phosphatidyl choline orally to animals fed an atherogenic diet and showed a preventive action (113). There is some debate about the mode of action of the phosphatidyl choline and other unsaturated compounds. Howard has suggested increased cholesterol ester hydrolase activity, or reduced ACAT production.

Blaton and Peters (114) suggest an increased activity of lipoprotein lipase as being important, whereas Adams and Abdulla (115) think that the role is to change the fatty acids esterifying cholesterol and that the resultant esters have a protective effect against atherosclerosis.

In 1961, Kritchevsky summarised the discussions of the Medicinal Division of the American Chemical Society on Hypercholesterolemic Agents (116). Even at that time the variety of substances available was considerable. There were drugs such as thyroxine and phenyl-substituted aliphatic acids that impaired cholesterol synthesis in liver slices. Nicotinic acid, which lowers all levels of serum lipids, also acts, most probably by affecting biosynthesis, though this is debatable. Other substances have been developed more recently; N-α-phenyl β-(p-tolyl) ethyl linoleamide (PTLA) has a remarkably hypercholesterolemic effect on rabbits. It is one of the many amides of linoleic acid that have been used. It also prevented the development of atherosclerosis in rabbits given as much as 1.6 g of cholesterol a day (117). The drug W-398 (benzyl-N-benzyl carbethoxyhydroxamate) is an effective hypocholesterolemic substance in rabbits and rats. It has an interesting mode of action by preventing the recirculation of labelled cholesterol after its uptake by the liver. However, the drug unfortunately has no such effect in monkeys or men (118). A number of other drugs behave in this way. For example IN-379 (1 Dimethyl aminoethyl 4-benzyl piperidine) is effective in preventing experimental atherosclerosis in rabbits and also promotes regression of induced lesions. However, it had no effect at all in the White Carneau pigeon (119). This emphasises again that, in the last analysis, man or possibly other primates are the only animals that are likely to provide meaningful results about human atherogenesis. Many other hypolipidemic-inducing drugs have been devised, and clofibrate is one of the best known of these. It will be considered under the title of *human experiments*.

Another approach to the task of lowering blood lipids is the employment of heparinlike substances. Grossman et al. reduced blood cholesterol and the extent of atheroma in cholesterol-fed rabbits by a heparitin sulphate with pronounced lipoprotein-lipase activating power (120). A similar effect was produced with another heparinoid laminarin sulphate in the cholesterol-fed rabbit (121). Heparin itself produces rather confusing results in different experimental animals. It is said to retard the development of atherosclerosis in rabbits (122), but continuous intravenous infusion of the drug for one year in dogs caused a 50 percent rise in serum cholesterol (123). The latter experiment clearly requires careful consideration in relation to long-term heparin therapy in man.

Another way of preventing deposition of lipid in the vessel wall might be to prevent the formation of complexes between calcium, lipoproteins, and other lipids in association with mucopolysaccharides. The parenteral administration of chelating agents such as the magnesium salt of ethylenediamine tetraacetic acid induced the reversal of plaques in the cholesterol-fed rabbit (124). This was associated with a reduction of the aortic calcium content. More direct evidence for the beneficial effects of chelation comes from the study of Wagner et al. (125) in the White Carneau pigeon. They fed cholesterol intermittently and produced advanced lesions; if these animals were injected with EHDP (ethane 1 hydroxy 1 1 diphosphonate) atherosclerosis regressed, and furthermore, the degree of mineralisation of the lesions was reduced. This occurred despite the absence of an effect on plasma lipids, calcium, or phosphorus, which suggested a direct effect on the vessel wall.

Using the concept of atherosclerosis as a proliferative, inflammatory response to injury, several agents, aimed at reducing the response, have been employed. The antihistamine chlorpheniramine is said to inhibit cholesterol-induced atherosclerosis in the rabbit but has no effect in the pig. Anti-inflammatory agents such as cortisone, phenylbutazone and amidopyrine have been shown to inhibit experimental atherosclerosis: aspirin, if anything, enhances development of lesions. It seems that most of these agents are usually effective in the rabbit, producing variable results in other species. This may be because they effect vascular permeability, which is an important pathogenic feature of cholesterol-induced atheroma in the rabbit (1). This view is supported by the demonstration of a protective effect of many steroids such as dexamethasone, 9-αfluorohydrocortisone, methylprednisolone and triamcinolone (126).

Drugs such as pyridinol carbamate (PDC), which antagonises bradykinin and, therefore, affects permeability, have no discernible effect in monkeys but are said to reduce cholesterol-induced atheroma in rabbits and chickens. A few workers have attempted to increase the permeability of the vessel wall to oxygen to mitigate the atherogenic effect of hypoxia. We have already seen that hyperoxia coupled with cholestyramine and oestrogen is anti-atherosclerotic (16). Attempts to change the levels of plasma proteins to improve oxygen diffusion have been unsuccessful as has the use of carotenoid compound, crocetin, which is also said to increase oxygen perfusion into the artery (1).

Experiments with Tissue Cultures

The first cardiovascular tissue culture conference was held in 1961. It was opened by O. J. Pollak, who emphasised the potential value of tissue culture in gaining an understanding of atherogenic mechanisms. Much subsequent work has reinforced that view. The problem of obtaining suitable experimental animals, particularly primates, also has encouraged the use of tissue culture methods. Pollak summarised his work and that of others in 1969 in a small monograph (127). Tissue culture results need careful critical evaluation. For example, it is not always easy to define the precise type of cell with which one is working, nor is it justifiable to assume that the cell does not change its characteristics on repeated culture. The methods used are mainly the culture of cells in layers or culture of slices of organs such as aorta. Even in 1961, when work was beginning to develop, workers were haggling over terminology of cells. Branwood reported the growth of aortic endothelial cells, but he also grew spindle cells, thought to be fibroblasts; inevitably, intermediate types of cells were named as well (128).

A variety of cells has been studied, endothelial cells having received much early attention. In later years, smooth muscle cells have been studied. Early work with endothelial cell cultures was often directed to their ability to synthesize lipids.

When it was found that the endothelial cells of White Carneau pigeons were less able to synthesize arachidonate from linoleate as compared to Show Racer pigeons, which have a much lesser tendency to develop atherosclerosis, it seemed that essential fatty acid deficiency was a likely atherogenic factor (129). These workers subsequently showed the presence of lipid vacuoles in the aortic cells of the White Carneau and postulated that they were derived from abnormal mitochondria that were deficient in ATPase activity. Similar vacuoles have been found in endothelial cells from human atheroma. However, lipid accumulation could not be induced by adding lipaemic serum to cultures of human aortic endothelium (130). Free fatty acids cause mitochondrial and lysosomal swelling and damage. Strangely, however, linoleate is more potent than stearate on cultured endothelial cells. The effect is more or less proportional to chain length and degree of saturation (132).

Heparinoid drugs such as laminaran sulphate have a significant depressive effect upon lipid synthesis by aortic cells given (^{14}C) acetate. Chondroitin polysulphate has a similar effect (132).

Attempts to elucidate the cause of the increased atherogenic risk of diabetes mellitus by a study of tissue cultures are as confusing as those in experimental animals. A study of the incorporation of (1-^{14}C) acetate and (1-^{14}C) oleic acid into the lipids of cultured human skin fibroblasts, derived from diabetics and controls, shows that cells from diabetics incorporate more acetate into cholesterol esters than do controls (132). On the other hand, studies of isolated animal aortas and tissue cultures of intimal cells have shown that insulin will enhance the incorporation of glucose into arterial lipids. Here again we have the situation where excess or lack of insulin seems to aggravate atherogenesis (133).

As previously mentioned, the smooth muscle cell has recently come to the forefront of discussions concerning atherogenesis. The discussion here will now turn to a study of smooth muscle cells in culture. Hyperlipidemic serum will cause esterified cholesterol and triglycerides to accumulate in these cells. In addition, hyperlipidemic serum will stimulate the proliferation of smooth muscle cells in explants of aortic tissue from monkeys. The greatest stimulant effect was achieved with low-density lipoproteins. The high-density lipoproteins had no effect (134). It is tempting to link these experimental results to the atherogenic potency of low-density lipoproteins in the experimental animal. Another stimulant effect on smooth muscle cell proliferation is observed when the serum of juvenile diabetics is added to cultures of rabbit aortic smooth muscle. A significant effect was produced using dialysed serum, and it appeared that the responsible factor was not lipid, glucose, amino acids, fructose, or ketones (135). The possibility remains that the growth factor may be the same as that described by Ross et al. from thrombocytes (136).

The combined effects of insulin and glucose on rat smooth muscle cells show that insulin has a stimulant effect on lipid synthesis. It probably works by stimulating the enzyme β-hydroxy-β-methyl glutamyl coenzyme A-reductase in that it stimulates the incorporation of acetate but not mevalonate into lipids. If used with high concentrations of glucose such as are found in uncontrolled diabetics, the synthesis of sterol is reduced (137). This finding is in accord with the lack of relationship between control of the diabetic state and the tendency to develop atherosclerotic disease (138).

Reversal of lipid accumulation has been shown in cultures of ascites cells and also using aortic smooth muscle cells. This release of membrane-bound cholesterol is achieved by human high-density lipoproteins added to the culture media. The specific component of the high-density lipoprotein seems to be its apolipoprotein (139). Pearson was able to show that reversal of lipid accumulation in rabbit aortic smooth muscle cells exposed to hyperlipemic serum could be achieved merely by removing the hyperlipemic stimulus. This loss of lipid occurred in as short a time as four days after withdrawing the hyperlipemic serum (140).

Synthesis of collagen, elastin, and precursor materials such as glycosaminoglycans is a function of arterial cells and is probably an important part of the atherosclerotic process. This has been studied in tissue culture preparations. Several workers have reported the synthesis of collagen and elastin by smooth muscle cells using biochemical, ultrastructural and conventional light microscopic techniques (141). Not only are glycosa-minoglycans involved in the processes of fibre synthesis by arterial cells, but they also have an interesting potential role in atherogenesis because they can bind low-density lipoproteins, which also have an atherogenic role. The effects of centrifugal stress on the synthesis of glycosaminoglycans (GAG) by pig aortic smooth muscle cells is interesting. This increases the synthesis of GAG and links with the observed role of hyperten-sive stress in promoting both atherosclerosis and the accumula-tion of GAG in vessel walls (142).

The relation between GAG synthesis and atherosclerosis is still, however, a controversial matter. Hyperlipemic serum will encourage the synthesis of collagen by embryonic filbroblasts and smooth muscle cells, but the effects are not always consis-tently reproducible in differing systems of cells.

There is still much to be done in defining the precise mode of action of various drugs on lipid and other metabolic pro-cesses in arterial cells. Tissue culture methods are well suited for such future experiments.

Experiments in Man

Many prospective attempts have been made to adjust the influence of various atherogenic factors in man. These involve dietary manipulation and the use of drugs to lower blood pres-sure, to dilate vessels, and to alter lipid metabolism. Few firm results are available at present because most of the prospective studies have been started recently, whereas atherosclerotic dis-ease and its complications are a slowly developing process. It takes as many as fifty years in most men before coronary artery disease begins to show any clinical effects.

Various "end points" are used to record coronary heart dis-ease. They include sudden death, infarction of the myocardium, and anginal pain, but only rarely is it possible, or ethical, to perform repeated angiography to assess the progress or regress of the disease. If angiography is not done then it is not possible to know why symptoms such as angina have improved in per-sons on a particular regime. A reduction of pain on exercise might be due to a real reduction in the size of existing atheroma by, for example, loss of lipid from the lesions. But equally, the phenomenon could be explained by the progressive development of a collateral circulation bypassing the narrowed main arteries. Collaterals may develop between branches of the main coronary arteries and also between coronary, bronchial, and internal mammary trunks.

Apart from hyperlipidemia and hypertension, there are few other factors that predict future development of coronary heart disease. Indeed, when all known factors are absent or minimal, myocardial infarction may still occur. Some have regarded arcus senilis, particularly in younger men, as a predictor of coronary heart disease. There is little support for this contention except when hyperlipidemia is also present (143).

An even more novel approach to the problem of determining the degree of vascular disease is an attempt to relate atheroma to dermal changes in skin biopsies. Bouisson et al. (144) postulate that age changes in skin develop *pari passu* with those in the aorta. The changes they describe have been graded from I to IV and consist of progressive loss of upper dermal elastic fibres with replacement by collagen, which gradually becomes more homogeneous and acellular. These alterations are accompanied by change in the lipid composition of the skin as well. This technique requires more thorough assessment.

At present, the approaches to regression in man have consisted of attempts to eliminate or reduce the various risk factors using several different criteria for the definition of coronary heart disease. Most surprisingly, the results are often inconclusive and even confusing. As with experimental animals, a lot of effort has been diverted towards changing the nature and quantity of dietary fats that are consumed. Wissler has often emphasised the atherogenic potency of the average American's diet and the reduced effect when the diet was made more "prudent" (145).

The primary efforts have been directed towards providing foods low in cholesterol content and containing high amounts of polyunsaturated fatty acids. In addition, the total caloric value of the diet has been reduced. Early efforts to achieve the compliance of the public resulted in a high "drop-out" rate. In more recent times, compliance is improved as a result of the progressive, sometimes ill-advised bombardment of people by every available broadcasting medium. However, even in 1976 in a sophisticated community in California, compliance was reached only as a result of intensive campaigns by mass media, courses of instruction, and personal visits. For example, men complied much less well if exposed to mass media alone. Better results were achieved by superadded intensive instruction (146). The result was a significant reduction in the intake of cholesterol and saturated fat by 20 to 40 percent, but it was much more difficult to persuade people to lower the dietary content of saturated fat and increase the intake of polyunsaturated fats. It was also difficult to get them to reduce weight and give up smoking.

A wide range of views has been expressed about the role of various fatty materials in the diet in relation to atherogenesis. They are summarised in Stern et al. (147). Yudkin related the intake of dietary fat to coronary thrombosis. He claimed that the effect held true up to a level of intake but also suggested that it may be the sterol content of the material and not the fat itself that might be atherogenic. Hugh Sinclair maintains that hypercholesterolemia is an expression of a deficiency of essential fatty acids, which can be corrected by diets rich in linoleic acid such as corn oil. Ancel Keys tested this hypothesis by feeding a variety of fats such as corn oil, butter fat, and sardine oil. He was not able to confirm that the level of serum cholesterol was simply related to the amount of essential fatty acids in the diet, nor was it related to the degree of unsaturation of the fatty acids. Kinsell and Sinclair challenged this work by saying that the precise composition of the fats used was not known. They reiterated the view that the cholesterol level was related to the degree of unsaturation of the dietary fats. Jones and Martin followed up by a study of fatty acids in patients with coronary artery disease and "controls," (author's quotation marks). They found no differences in phospholipids in the two groups. However, age-matched controls in this sort of case are clearly meaningless. The control may have just as severe coronary artery disease but symptoms have not yet become manifest.

The extreme end of the spectrum is seen in hypercholesterolemic xanthomatosis. Attempts to treat this by a diet rich in corn oil have had some measure of success. After four months, cholesterol levels fell and some of the xanthomas regressed. Angina, however, in some cases was unaffected (148).

An ambitious project to study the effects of polyunsaturated fats in the diet was mounted by the Anti-Coronary Club in the late 1950s. There were 814 test subjects and 463 males of comparable age. The men in both groups were clinically free of coronary heart disease. The study ran for almost six years. A significant drop in the incidence of coronary heart disease was found in the experimental group. In men forty to forty-nine years old, there was one new coronary event in the experimental group and four in the controls. There was, however, no difference in the fifty to fifty-nine year olds in either group (149).

Another large project, the Coronary Drug Project, has been in progress in the United States. It involves 8,341 men aged thirty to sixty-four years on entry to the study. The work was done in fifty-three centres throughout the United States. All patients before entry into the study had suffered one or more cardiac infarcts. There were three basic objectives: to observe the efficiency of four different drugs on serum lipids, to study the course and prognosis of coronary heart disease, and to learn about the problems of control of multicentre trials. The drugs used were oestrogens, clofibrate, dextrothyroxine, and nicotinic acid. One thing clearly emerges from this work to date, namely that such multifactorial trials are very difficult to interpret (150).

Apparently, the maximum reduction of serum cholesterol that can be achieved by dietary manipulation alone is 20 percent. If this reduction had been maintained for the entire life of the individual then it might be expected that the incidence of coronary heart disease would be reduced by almost 40 percent. The effect of shorter periods of dietary modification, however, is not known.

Many drugs have been used to augment the hypocholesterolemic effects of dietary modifications. Of these, clofibrate is the most widely known and used. It has many actions, but whether any of these are beneficial in coronary heart disease is still unclear. For example, it causes a fall of plasma triglyceride levels probably by increasing tissue utilisation of triglycerides. However, the relationship between plasma triglycerides and coronary heart disease is unclear. They are probably of no significance. Clofibrate also lowers levels of plasma free fatty acids. The effects on serum cholesterol are much less definite. It is also said to decrease fibrinogen levels, enhance fibrinolysis, and reduce platelet stickiness. In more recent times it is purported to raise the levels of high-density lipoproteins. In regard to the experimental studies that we have discussed previously, it might be considered that clofibrate is the universal panacea for atherosclerotic heart disease and its complications.

A large-scale trial of this drug was proposed in Scotland and Newcastle upon Tyne, and the results were reported in 1971 (151). About 1,214 patients were involved, and the results were rather disappointing. The mortality from myocardial infarction was the same in the group receiving clofibrate and in the controls. A curious result emerged from this trial: those patients who had entered the trial with angina pectoris were less likely to die of myocardial infarction when given clofibrate than those who had no angina. It could well be that clofibrate has another pharmacological action, which is independent of its lipid-lowering properties. A study by Krasmo and Kidera (152) supports this view. They found that clofibrate reduced the incidence of myocardial infarction in men free of coronary heart disease at the start of the trial. This was despite the considerable variation of blood lipid levels among the treated group. The role of clofibrate in the management of ischaemic heart disease still remains problematical. The situation has changed little since the publication of a double issue of the *Journal of Atherosclerosis Research* devoted to studies of clofibrate in 1963 (153). The search for a potent hypocholesterolemic drug with few side effects goes on, and several new drugs have been reported recently.

Another large group of substances has been employed to impede the absorbtion of cholesterol from the gut. These vary from dietary fibre, ion exchange resins such as cholestyramine and colestipol and sulphaguanidine. All have a cholesterol-lowering effect and, in conjunction with other forms of therapy, are liable to form an important part of the regime for preventing or regressing atherosclerotic disease.

Ileal bypass is the most effective means of lowering serum cholesterol and lipoproteins in man. Of course, it can only be used in extreme examples of hypercholesterolemia with a high risk of developing coronary disease. There are several undesirable features, such as intractable diarrhoea, that may follow the operation. However, a reduction of cholesterol by 50 percent has been achieved by this operation; furthermore, tendon xanthomas have regressed after it has been done. In such patients, serial coronary arteriograms have shown no increase in lesions over the space of two years. The whole subject of ileal bypass is well reviewed by Henry Buchwald (154).

At present, hypotensive therapy is usually instituted only after the patient has had some clinical event. There is considerable resistance among doctors and patients to allow the treatment of symptomless hypertension. It follows that the institution of therapy is liable to be in middle age when coronary artery disease might be well established and severely occlusive. The proper study of the action of hypotensives can only be done when early treatment is started and continued for some years. From all the evidence available in experimental animals, it is likely to show some regressive or preventive effect on coronary heart disease. Another important matter in this context is to be sure that the hypertension is indeed properly controlled. Sporadic readings of blood pressure at ill-assorted times are no measure. Patients need to be taught to measure their pressures and to log the results for a few months. The experiment of the effect of hypotensives on human coronary disease has not yet been done properly.

Further time is also needed to assess the effects of smoking on coronary disease. There does seem to be a relationship between cigarette smoking and the development of coronary artery disease in studies of British civil servants, among Negroes in the United States and in Japanese men and women. These are some of the studies that have been done and show that the risk of dying of coronary heart disease for all smokers is one and one-half to two and one-half times that of nonsmokers. For heavy smokers, the risk is about three and one-half times. It is particularly interesting that the mortality from coronary heart disease for women aged thirty-five to forty-four increased by more than a third between 1958 and 1970. During that period, the average weekly consumption of cigarettes in the United Kingdom doubled in women aged sixteen to twenty-four and increased 35 percent in all women.

In 1976, Doll and Peto (155) published the results of their study of the smoking habits of British doctors, which was started in 1951. The ratio of the death rate among cigarette smokers to lifelong nonsmokers was 2:1 for men under seventy years of age. This suggests that about half of the deaths in smokers are due to their smoking. Not all causes of death are, of course, due to coronary heart disease. Many of the doctors gave up smoking after 1951, and the mortality rate fell from the fourth to the twentieth year of the study by 28 percent in men under sixty-five years of age.

The results of this human experiment seem to be conclusive though studies in all countries, for example in Yugoslavia, have not always related smoking and coronary heart disease. A clear relationship does exist between smoking or the inhalation of carbon monoxide and the aggravation of anginal pain. Inhalation of 50 ppm of CO caused a rise of venous carboxyhaemo- globin to about 2.9 percent. Such a concentration, which is often found in densely populated urban areas, aggravated angina pectoris (156). Other workers have related the level of blood carboxyhaemoglobin (COHb) to cardiovascular disease risk. In the age group thirty to sixty-nine, persons with COHb levels of 50 percent or more were twenty-one times more likely to develop ischaemic heart disease as compared to persons of comparable age, sex, and smoking history where COHb levels were less than 3 percent (157).

Most of these human experiments, as is the case with animal experiments, have not cast much light on the fundamental causes of atherosclerotic disease; they only serve to emphasise those things that aggravate the conditions. One of the most fundamental experiments was the transplantation of the heart of a twenty-four-year-old man into a man of fifty-eight years. Twenty months later the transplanted heart showed severe oc- clusive coronary artery disease (158). The author of this paper suggested that the high blood cholesterol of the recipient (300 mgm/100 ml) was the responsible factor. This is most unlikely to be true. Much more reasonable is the concept of an immune response in the artery wall leading to immune complex formation, platelet aggregation, and subsequent atherosclerosis. This important experiment underlines the role of immune responses and platelets in atherogenesis. Attempts to prevent platelet aggregation in the arteries of transplanted organs have been moderately successful. A variety of drugs has been used including dipyridamole, which is an inhibitor of platelet aggregation. For this and other reasons, cardiac transplantation is likely to be a useful procedure in certain selected areas.

References

1. Gresham, G. A.: Is atheroma a reversible lesion. *Atherosclerosis, 23:*379, 1976.
2. Constantinides, P. and Robinson, M.: Ultrastructural injury of arterial endothelium. *Arch Pathol, 88:*99, 1969.
3. Astrup, P. and Kjeldsen, K.: Carbon monoxide, smoking and atherosclerosis. *Med Clin North Am, 58:*2, 1974.
4. Miller, G. J. and Miller, N. E.: Plasma-high-density lipoprotein concentration and development of ischaemic heart disease. *Lancet, i:*16, 1975.
5. Davies, D. F.: Hypothesis — An immunological view of atherosclerosis. *J Atheroscler Res, 10:*253, 1969.
6. Van Winkle, M. and Levy, L.: Effect of removal of cholesterol diet upon serum-sickness-cholesterol induced atherosclerosis. *J Exp Med, 128:*497, 1968.
7. Horlick, L. and Katz, L. N.: Regression of atherosclerotic lesions on cessation of cholesterol feeding in the chick. *J Lab Clin Med, 34:*1427, 1949.
8. Anitschkow, N.: Uber die Ruckbildunsvorgange Bei Der Experimentellen Atherosklerose. *Verh Dtsh Ges Pathol, 23:*473, 1928.
9. Schuler, W.: Discussion in *J Atheroscler Res, 2:*149, 1962.
10. Weber, G., Fabbrini, P., Capaccioli, E., and Resi, L.: Repair of early cholesterol-induced aortic lesions. *Atherosclerosis, 22:*565, 1975.
11. Bortz, W. M.: Reversibility of atherosclerosis in cholesterol-fed rabbits. *Circ Res, 22:*135, 1968.
12. Björkerud, S. and Bondjers, G.: Repair responses and tissue lipid after experimental injury to the artery. *Ann NY Acad Sci, 275:*180, 1976.
13. Constantinides, P., Booth, J., and Carlson, G.: Production of advanced atherosclerosis in rabbit. *Arch Pathol,70:*712, 1960.
14. Adams, C. W. M., Morgan, R. S., and Bayliss, O. B.: No regression of

atheroma over one year in rabbits previously fed on cholesterol enriched diet. *Atherosclerosis, 18:*429, 1973.

15. Loustalot, P. and Hess, R.: Delayed spontaneous regression of experimental aortic lipidosis in the rat. *J Atheroscler Res, 3:*288, 1963.

16. Vesselinovitch, D., Wissler, R. W., Fisher-Dzoga, K., Hughes, R., and Dubien, L.: Regression of atherosclerosis in rabbits Part I *Atherosclerosis, 19:*259, 1974.

17. Maruffo, C. A. and Portman, O. W.: Nutritional control of coronary artery atherosclerosis in the squirrel monkey. *J Atheroscler Res, 8:*237, 1968.

18. Armstrong, M. L. and Megan, M. B.: Lipid deposition in atheromatous coronary arteries in rhesus monkeys after regression diets. *Circ Res, 30:*675, 1972.

19. Eggen, D. A., Strong, J. P., Newman, W. P., Catsulis, C., Malcolm, G. T., and Kokatnur, M. G.: Regression of the diet-induced fatty streaks in rhesus monkeys. *Lab Invest, 31:*294, 1974.

20. Armstrong, M. L. and Megan, M. B.: Arterial fibrous proteins in cynomolgus monkeys after atherogenic and regression regimes (Abst). *Circulation (Suppl 4), 43:*41, 1973.

21. Kokatnur, M. G., Malcolm, G. T., Eggen, D. A., and Strong, J. P.: Depletion of aortic cholesterol in rhesus monkeys. *Atherosclerosis, 21:*195, 1975.

22. Tucker, C. G., Catsulis, C., Strong, J. P., and Eggen, D. A.: Regression of early cholesterol-induced aortic lesions in rhesus monkeys. *Am J Pathol, 65:*493, 1971.

23. Strong, J. P., Eggen, D. A., and Stary, H. C.: Reversibility of fatty streaks in rhesus monkeys. In *Primates in Medicine.* Basel, Karger, *9:*1975.

24. Daoud, A. S., Jarmolych, J., Augustyn, J. M., Fritz, K. E., Singh, J. K., and Lee, K. T.: Regression of advanced atherosclerosis in swine. *Arch Path Lab Med, 100:*372, 1976.

25. DePalma, R. G., Hubay, C. A., Insull, W., Robinson, A. G., and Hartman, P. H.: Progression and regression of experimental atherosclerosis. *Surg Gynecol Obstet, 131:*633, 1970.

26. Prichard, R. W., Clarkson, T. B., Goodman, H. O., and Lofland, H. B.: Coronary atherosclerosis. *Arch Pathol, 81:*292, 1966.

27. McCance, R. A.: The bearing of early nutrition on later development. *Proc 6th Int Congr Nutr,* 74, 1963.

28. Liebman, J., Leash, A., Benyo, R., and Wallace, W. M.: Effects of early underfeeding on weight of White Carneau pigeon. *Atherosclerosis, 11:*439, 1970.

29. Malmros, H. and Wigand, G.: Atherosclerosis and deficiency of essential fatty acids. *Lancet, ii:*749, 1959.

30. Hill, E. G., Warmanen, E. L., Hayes, H., and Holman, R. T.: Effects of essential fatty acid deficiency in young swine. *Proc Soc Expt Biol Med, 96:*274, 1957.

31. Morin, R. J., Bernick, S., and Alfin-Slater, R. B.: Effects of essential fatty

acids on atheromas. *J Atheroscler Res, 4:*387, 1964.

32. Gresham, G. A.: The use of primates in cardiovascular research. In Bourne, G. (Ed.): *Nonhuman Primates in Medical Research.* New York, Acad Pr, 1973, p. 234.

33. Pick, R., Stamler, J., and Katz, L. N.: Effects of high protein intake on cholesterolemia and atherogenesis in growing and mature chickens fed high-fat, high-cholesterol diets. *Circ Res, 7:*866, 1959.

34. Kokatnur, M., Rand, N. T., Kummerow, F. A., and Scott, H. M.: Effect of dietary protein and fat on changes of serum cholesterol in mature birds. *J Nutr, 64:*177, 1968.

35. Pick, R., Savitri, J., Katz, L. N., and Johnson, P · Fffect of dietary protein level on regression of cholesterol-induced hypercholesterolemia and atherosclerosis of cockerels. *J Atheroscler Res, 5:*16, 1965.

36. Mann, G. V.: Sterol metabolism in monkeys. Dietary cholesterol and protein in maintenance of sterol compensation. *Circ Res, 9:*838, 1961.

37. Polcák, J., Melichar, F., Ševelová, D., Dvořák, I., and Skálová, M.: Effect of meat in diet on experimental atherosclerosis in rabbits. *J Atheroscler Res, 5:*174, 1965.

38. Saraswathi, D. and Kurup, P. A.: Hypolipedemic activity of *Phaseolus mungo* (blackgram) in rats fed high fat high cholesterol diet. *Atherosclerosis, 15:*223, 1972.

39. Prema, L. and Kurup, P. A.: Effect of protein fractions from *Cajanus cajan* (redgram) and *Dolichos biflorus* (horsegram) on the serum, liver and aortic lipid levels in rats fed a high fat high cholesterol diet. *Atherosclerosis, 18:*369, 1973.

40. McGill, H. C., Frank, M. H., and Geer, J. C.: Aortic lesions in hypertensive monkeys. *Arch Pathol, 71:*96, 1961.

41. Altschul, R.: In *Selected Studies on Arteriosclerosis.* Springfield, Thomas, 1950.

42. Roffo, A. H.: Egg-plant *(Solanum melongena L.)* in decholesterolization. *Yale J Biol Med, 18:*25, 1945.

43. Grant, W. C.: Influence of avocados on serum cholesterol. *Proc Soc Exp Biol Med, 104:*45, 1960.

44. Cookson, F. B., Altschul, R., and Fedoroff, S.: The effects of alfalfa on serum cholesterol and in modifying or preventing cholesterol induced atherosclerosis in rabbits. *J Atheroscler Res, 7:*69, 1967.

45. Howard, A. N., Gresham, G. A., Jones, D., and Jennings, I. W.: Prevention of rabbit atherosclerosis by soya bean meal. *J Atheroscler Res, 5:*330, 1965.

46. Dixon, K. C.: Deposition of globular lipids in arterial cells in relation to anoxia. *Am J Pathol, 39:*65, 1969.

47. Sackett, D. L. Gibson, R. W., Brass, I. D., and Pickren, J. W.: Relation between aortic atherosclerosis and the use of cigarettes and alcohol. *N Engl J Med, 279:*1413, 1968.

48. Strong, J. P., Richards, M. L., McGill, H. C. Jr., Eggen, D. A., and McMurray, M. T.: On the association of cigarette smoking with

coronary and aortic atherosclerosis. *J Atheroscler Res,* 10:303, 1969.
49. Strong, J. P. and Richards, M. L.: Cigarette smoking and atherosclerosis in autopsied men. *Atherosclerosis,* 23:451, 1976.
50. Garbarsch, C., Matthiessen, M. E., Helin, P., and Lorenzen, L.: Arteriosclerosis and hypoxia Part I. *J Atheroscler Res,* 9:283, 1969.
51. Helin, P., Lorenzen, I., Garbarsch, C., and Matthiessen, M. E.: Arteriosclerosis and hypoxia Part 2. *J Atheroscler Res,* 9:295, 1969.
52. Helin, G., Helin, P., and Lorenzen, I.: Aortic glycosaminoglycans in arteriosclerosis. *Atherosclerosis,* 12:235, 1970.
53. Yant, W. P., Chornyak, J., Schrenk, H. H., Patty, F. A., and Sayers, R. R.: Studies in Asphyxia (Public Health Bulletin No 211) Washington, 1934.
54. Wanstrup, J., Kjeldsen, K., and Astrup, P.: Acceleration of spontaneous intimal-subintimal changes in rabbit aorta by a prolonged moderate carbon monoxide exposure. *Acta Pathol Microbiol Scand,* 75:353, 1969.
55. Kjeldsen, K., Astrup, P., and Wanstrup, J.: Intimal changes in rabbit aorta after CO exposure. *Atherosclerosis,* 16:67, 1972.
56. Elemér, G., Kerényi, T., and Jellinek, H.: Scanning and transmission electron microscopic studies in post-ischaemic endothelial lesions following recirculation. *Atherosclerosis,* 24:219, 1976.
57. Davies, R. F., Topping, D. L., and Turner, D. M.: The effect of intermittent carbon monoxide exposure on experimental atherosclerosis in the rabbit. *Atherosclerosis,* 24:527, 1976.
58. Astrup, P.: Some physiological and pathological effects of moderate carbon monoxide exposure. *Br Med J,* 2:447, 1972.
59. Thomsen, H. K.: Carbon monoxide induced atherosclerosis in primates. *Atherosclerosis,* 20:233, 1974.
60. Turner, D. M. and Topping, D. L.: The effects of tobacco smoke and some of its constituents on triglyceride secretion in the squirrel monkey. *Res Commun Chem Pathol Pharmacol,* 12:85, 1975.
61. Armitage, A. K., Davies, R. F., and Turner, D. M.: The effects of carbon monoxide on the development of atherosclerosis in the White Carneau pigeon. *Atherosclerosis,* 23:333, 1976.
62. Lindy, S., Turto, H., Uitto, J., Garbarsch, C., Helin, P., and Lorenzen, L.: The effect of chronic hypoxia on lactate dehydrogenase in rabbit arterial wall *Atherosclerosis,* 20:295, 1974.
63. Sarma, J. S. M., Tillmanns, H., Ikeda, S., and Bing, R. J.. The effect of carbon monoxide on lipid metabolism of human coronary arteries. *Atherosclerosis,* 22:193, 1975.
64. Howard, C. F. and Bonnett, L.: Effects of hypoxic and aerobic incubation on lipogenesis from (^{14}C) glucose in sections of normal and atherosclerotic aorta from the rabbit. *Atherosclerosis,* 18:469, 1973.
65. Moschos, C. B., Ahmed, S. S., Kamalesh, L., and Regan, T. J.: Chronic smoking in an animal model. *Atherosclerosis,* 23:437, 1976.
66. Frith, C. H., McMurty, I. F., Alexander, A. F., and Will, D. H.: Influence of hypertension and hypoxemia on arterial biochemistry and

morphology in swine. *Atherosclerosis, 20:*189, 1974.
67. Altschul, R. and Herman, I. H.: Influence of oxygen inhalation on cholesterol metabolism. *Arch Biochem, 51:*308, 1954.
68. Kjeldsen, K., Astrup, P., Wanstrup, J.: Reversal of rabbit atherosclerosis by hyperoxia. *J Atheroscler Res, 10:*173, 1969.
69. Prior, J. T. and Ziegler, D. D.: Regression of experimental atherosclerosis. *Arch Pathol, 80:*50, 1965.
70. Vesselinovitch, D., Wissler, R. W., Fisher-Dzoga, K., Hughes, R., and Dubien, L.: Regression of atherosclerosis in rabbits. *Atherosclerosis, 19:*259, 1974.
71. DePalma, R. G., Koletsky, S., Bellon, E. R., and Insull, W., Jr.: Failure of regression of atherosclerosis in dogs with moderate cholesterolemia. *Atherosclerosis, 27:*297, 1977.
72. Stamler, J.: Current status of knowledge on oestrogen treatment of hyperlipidemia and atherosclerotic disease. In Casdorph, H. R. (Ed.): *Treatment of the Hyperlipidemic State.* Springfield, Thomas, 1971, p. 370.
73. London, W. T., Rosenberg, S. E., Draper, J. W., and Almy, T. P.: The effect of oestrogen on atherosclerosis. A post-mortem study. *Ann Intern Med, 55:*63, 1961.
74. Gresham, G. A. and Howard, A. N.: The independent production of atherosclerosis and thrombosis in the rat. *Br J Exp Pathol, 41:*395, 1960.
75. Stamler, J., Pick, R., and Katz, L. N.: Saturated and unsaturated fats. Effects on cholesterolemia and atherogenesis in chicks on high-cholesterol diets. *Circ Res, 398:*1959.
76. Stamler, J., Pick, R., and Katz, L. N.: In Pincus, G.: *Hormones and Atherosclerosis.* New York, Acad Pr, 1959, p. 173.
77. Stamler, J., Pick, R., and Katz, L. N.: Effects of desoxycorticosterone acetate on cholesterolemia, blood pressure and atherogenesis in chicks. *Circulation, 4:*262, 1951.
78. Peters, N. and Hales, C. N.: Plasma insulin concentrations in myocardial infarction. *Lancet, i:*1144, 1965.
79. Gertler, M. M., Leetman, H. E., Saluste, E., Welsh, J. J., Rusk, H. A., Covalt, D. A., and Rosenberger, J.: Carbohydrate insulin and lipid inter-relationship in ischaemic vascular disease. *Geriatrics, 25:*134, 1970.
80. Sloan, J. S., Mackay, J. S., and Sheridan, B.: Glucose tolerance and insulin response in atherosclerosis. *Br Med J, 4:*586, 1970.
81. Stout, R. W.: Insulin-stimulated lipogenesis in arterial tissue in relation to diabetes and atheroma. *Lancet, ii:*702, 1968.
82. Stout, R. W. and Vallance-Owen, J.: Insulin and atheroma. *Lancet, i:*1078, 1969.
83. Stamler, J. and Katz, L. N.: The effect of pancreatectomy on lipemia, tissue lipidosis and atherogenesis in chicks. *Circulation, 4:*255, 1951.
84. Pick, R., Stamler, J., Rodbard, S., and Katz, L. N.: Inhibition of

coronary athcrosclerosis by oestrogens in cholesterol-fed chicks. *Circ Res, 6:*276, 1952.

85. Pick, R., Stamler, J., and Katz, L. N.: Susceptibility of the ovariectomized hen to cholesterol-induced coronary atherogenesis. *Circ Res, 5:*515, 1957.

86. Katz, L. N. and Pick, R.: Experimental atherosclerosis in chickens. *J Atheroscler Res, i:*93, 1961.

87. Chobanian, A. V.: Effects of sex hormones on phospholipid R.N.A. and protein metabolism in the arterial intima. *J Atheroscler Res, 8:*763, 1968.

88. Gore, I., Iwanaga, Y., and Gore, H.: Inhibition of dietary atherosclerosis in rabbits by norethynodrel. *J Atheroscler Res, 7:*361, 1967.

89. Kroman, H. S., Bender, S. R., Brest, A. N., and Moskovitz, M. L.: The inter-relationship of blood lipids and estrogens. *J Atheroscler Res, 6:*247, 1966.

90. Phillips, G. B.: Evidence for hyperoestrogenaemia as a risk factor for myocardial infarction in men. *Lancet, ii:*14, 1976.

91. Stern, M. P., Brown, B. W., Haskell, W. L., Farquhar, J. W., Wehrle, C. L., and Wood, P. D. S.: Cardiovascular risk and use of oestrogens or oestrogen-prostagen combinations. *JAMA, 811:*235, 1976.

92. Renaud, S.: Thrombosis and atherosclerosis prevention by estrogens in hyperlipidemic rats. *Atherosclerosis, 12:*467, 1970.

93. Levy, L.: A form of immunological atherosclerosis. In Luzio, N. R. D. and Paoletti, R. (Eds.): *Advances in Experimental Medicine and Biology,* vol. 1. New York, Plenum Pr, 1967, p. 426.

94. Van Winkle, M. and Levy, L.: Effect of removal of cholesterol diet upon serum sickness — Cholesterol-induced atherosclerosis. *J Exp Med, 128:*497, 1968.

95. Howard, A. N., Patelski, J., Bowyer, D. E., and Gresham, G. A.: Atherosclerosis induced in hypercholesterolemic baboons, by immunological injury; and the effects of intravenous polyunsaturated phosphatidyl choline. *Atherosclerosis, 14:*17, 1971.

96. Biozzi, G., Mené, G., and Ovary, Z.: L'histamine et la granulopexie de l'endothelium vasculaire. *Rev Immunol (Paris), 12:*320, 1948.

97. Gell, P. G. H. and Coombs, R. R. A.: Clinical Aspects of Immunology. Oxford and Edinburgh, 1968, p. 725.

98. Cochrane, C. G.: Studies on the localisation of circulating antigen antibody complexes and other macromolecules in vessels. *J Exp Med, 118:*503, 1963.

99. Haimovici, H. and Maier, N.: Role of arterial tissue susceptibility in experimental canine atherosclerosis. *J Atheroscler Res, 6:*62, 1966.

100. Fisher, E. R. and Fisher, B.: Effect of induced atherosclerosis on fresh and lyophilised aortic homografts in rabbits. *Surgery, 40:*530, 1956.

101. Bowyer, D. E., Dunn, D., and Gresham, G. A.: Production of advanced atheromatous lesions in an allografted segment in normocholesterolemic rabbit. In Schettler, F. G. and Weizel, A.:

Atherosclerosis III Proceedings of the Third International Symposium. Berlin, Springer-Verlag, 1974, p. 348.

102. Gerö, S.: Allergy and autoimmune factors. In Schettler, F. G. and Boyd, G. S. (Eds.): *Atherosclerosis.* Amsterdam, Elsevier, 1969, p. 455.

103. Tromp, S. W.: *Medical Biometerology.* Amsterdam, Elsevier, 1963, p. 506.

104. Davies, D. F.: Hypothesis — an immunological view of atherogenesis. *J Atheroscler Res, 10:*253, 1969.

105. Rounds, D. E., Boother, J., and Guerrero, R. R.: Consideration of atherosclerotic plaques as benign neoplasms. *Atherosclerosis, 25:*183, 1976.

106. Berger, F. M., Vaniitallie, T. B., Tennent, D. M., and Stebrell, W. H.: Effect of anion exchange resin on serum cholesterol in man. *Proc Soc Exp Biol Med, 102:*676, 1959.

107. Parkinson, T. M., Gundersen, K., and Nelson, N. A.: Effects of colestipol (U-26, 597A), a new bile acid sequestrant on serum lipids in experimental animals and man. *Atherosclerosis, 11:*531, 1970.

108. Buchwald, H.: The effect of ileal bypass on atherosclerosis and hypercholesterolemia in the rabbit. *Surgery, 58:*22, 1965.

109. Scott, H. W., Jr., Stephenson, S. E. Jr., Younger, R., Carlisle, B. B. and Turney, S. W.: Prevention of experimental atherosclerosis by ileal bypass. *Ann Surg, 163:*795, 1966.

110. Flynn, K. J., Schumacher, J. F., Ravi Subbiah, M. T., and Kottke, B. A.: The effect of ileal bypass on sterol balance and plasma cholesterol in the White Carneau pigeon. *Atherosclerosis, 24:*75, 1976.

111. Hurwitz, S., Bar, A., Katz, L. N., Sklan, D., and Budowski, P.: Absorptional secretion of fatty acids and bile acids in the intestine of the laying fowl. *J Nutr, 103:*543, 1973.

112. Howard, A. N. and Patelski, J.: Hydrolysis and synthesis of aortic cholesterol esters in atherosclerotic baboons. *Atherosclerosis, 20:*225, 1974.

113. Samo Chowiec, L., Kadlubowska, D., and Rózewicka, L.: Investigations in experimental atherosclerosis Part I. The effects of phosphatidyl choline (E.P.L.) on experimental atherosclerosis in white rats. *Atherosclerosis, 23:*305, 1976.

114. Blaton, B. and Peeters, H.: Effect of unsaturated phosphatidyl choline on the lipoprotein lipase activity in vivo. In Schettler, F. G. and Weizel, A. (Eds.): *Atherosclerosis III.* Berlin, Springer-Verlag, 1974, p. 565.

115. Adams, C. W. M. and Abdulla, Y. H.: Polyunsaturated phospholipids and experimental atherosclerosis. In *Phospholipids.* Stuttgart, George Thieme, 1972, p. 44.

116. Kritchevsky, D.: Hypocholesteremic agents. *J Atheroscler Res, 1:*345, 1961.

117. Nakatani, H., Aono, S., Suzuki, Y., Fukushima, H., Nakamuray, Y., and Toki, K.: The effect of N-(α phenyl-β-(p-tolyl) ethyl) linoleamide

on experimental atherosclerosis in rabbits. *Atherosclerosis, 12:*307, 1970.

118. Douglas, J. F., Ludwig, B. J., Margolin, S., and Berger, F. M.: Hypocholesterolemic action of W398. *J Atheroscler Res, 6:*90, 1966.
119. Kottke, B. A., Juergens, J. L., Zollman, P. E.: Effect of 1 Dimethyl-aminoethyl-4 Benzylpiperidine (IN 379) on aortic atherosclerosis of White Carneau pigeons. *J Atheroscler Res, 6:*87, 1966.
120. Grossman, B. J., Cifonelli, J. A., and Ozoa, A. K.: Inhibition of atherosclerosis in cholesterol-fed rabbits by a heparitin sulphate. *Atherosclerosis, 13:*103, 1971.
121. Besterman, E. M. M.: Laminarin sulphate and experimental atherosclerosis. *Atherosclerosis, 12:*85, 1970.
122. Constantinides, P., Szasz, G., and Harden, F.: Retardation of atheromatosis and adrenal enlargement by heparin in the rabbit. *Arch Pathol, 56:*36, 1963.
123. Blackshear, P. J., Rhode, T. D., Varco, R. L., and Buchwald, H.: The effect of continuous heparin infusion for one year on serum cholesterol and triglyceride concentrations in the dog. *Atherosclerosis, 26:*23, 1977.
124. Wartman, A., Lampe, T. L., McCann, D. S., and Boyle, A. J.: Plaque reversal with Mg. E.D.T.A. in experimental atherosclerosis. *J Atheroscler Res, 7:*331, 1967.
125. Wagner, W. D., Clarkson, T. B., and Foster, J.: Contrasting effects of ethane-1-Hydroxy-1, 1-Diphosphonate (EHDP) on the regression of two types of dietary atherosclerosis. *Atherosclerosis, 27:*419, 1977.
126. Bailey, J. M. and Butler, J.: Anti-inflammatory drugs in experimental atherosclerosis. *Atherosclerosis, 17:*515, 1973.
127. Pollak, O. J.: *Tissue Cultures.* Basel, S. Karger, 1969.
128. Branwood, A. W.: Cardiovascular tissue culture. *J Atheroscler Res, 1:*358, 1961.
129. Smith, S. C., Strout, R. G., Dunlop, W. R., and Smith, E. C.: Fatty acids of cultured aortic cells from two breeds of pigeons. *J Atheroscler Res, 5:*379, 1965.
130. Myasinikov, A. L., Block, Y. E., and Pavlov, V. M.: Influence of lipemic serums of patients with atherosclerosis. *J Atheroscler Res, 6:*224, 1966.
131. Acosta, D. and Wenzel, D. G.: Injury produced by free fatty acids to lysosomes and mitochondria in cultured heart muscle and endothelial cells. *Atherosclerosis, 20:*417, 1974.
132. Murata, K.: Suppression of lipid synthesis in cultured aortic cells by laminarin sulphate. *J Atheroscler Res, 10:*371, 1969.
133. Cooper, J. T. and Goldstein, S.: De novo synthesis of lipids and incorporation of oleic acid into cultured human fibroblasts from diabetics and normal controls. *Atherosclerosis, 20:*41, 1974.
134. Mahler, R. and Parkes, A. B.: Fat synthesis in cultures of cells of arterial intima. *Eur J Clin Invest, 1:*137, 1970.
135. Fischer-Dzoga, K. and Wissler, R. W.: Stimulation of Proliferation in

stationary primary cultures of monkey aortic smooth muscle cells. *Atherosclerosis, 24:*515, 1976.

136. Ledet, T.: Growth of rabbit aortic smooth muscle cells in serum from patients with juvenile diabetes. *Acta Pathol Microbiol Scand Sect A, 84:*508, 1976.

137. Ross, R., Glomset, J., Karyya, B., and Harker, L.: A platelet dependent serum factor that stimulated the proliferation of arterial smooth muscle cells in vitro. *Proc Natl Acad Sci USA, 71:*1207, 1974.

138. Stout, R. W.: The effect of insulin and glucose on sterol synthesis in cultured rat arterial smooth muscle cells. *Atherosclerosis, 27:*271, 1977.

139. Stout, R. W., Bierman, E. L., and Brunzell, J. D.: Atherosclerosis and disorders of lipid metabolism in diabetes. In Vallance-Owen, J. (Ed.): *Diabetes — Its Physiological and Biochemical Basis.* Lancaster, MTP Press, 1975, p. 125.

140. Stein, Y., Glangeaud, M. C., Fainaru, M., and Stein, O.: The removal of cholesterol from aortic smooth muscle cells in culture and Landschutz ascites cells by fractions of human high density lipoproteins. *Acta Biochem Biophys, 380:*106, 1975.

141. Pearson, J. D.: Lipid metabolism in cultured aortic smooth muscle cells and comparison with other cell types. *Atherosclerosis, 25:*205, 1976.

142. Boissel, J. P., Bourdillon, M. C., Loire, R., and Crouzet, B.: Histological arguments for collagen and elastin synthesis by primary cultures of rat aortic media cells. *Atherosclerosis, 25:*107, 1976.

143. Merrilees, M. J., Merrilees, M. A., Birnbaum, P. S., Scott, P. J., and Flint, M. H.: The effect of centrifugal force on glycosaminoglycan production by aortic smooth muscle cells in culture. *Atherosclerosis, 27:*259, 1977.

144. McAndrew, G. M. and Ogston, D.: Arcus senilis and coronary artery disease. *Am Heart J, 70:*838, 1965.

145. Boissou, H., Pieraggi, M. Th., Julian, M., Buscail, I., Douste-Blazy, L., Latorre, E., and Charlet, J. P.: Identifying arteriosclerosis and aortic atheromatosis by skin biopsy. *Atherosclerosis, 19:*449, 1974.

146. Wissler, R. W. and Vesselinovitch, D.: The effect of feeding various dietary fats on the development and regression of hypercholesterolemia and atherosclerosis. In Sirtori, C., Ricci, G., and Gorinin, S. (Eds.): *Diet and Atherosclerosis.* New York, Plenum Pr, 1975.

147. Stern, M. P., Farquhar, J. W., Maccoby, N., and Russell, S. H.: Results of a two-year health education campaign on dietary behaviour. *Circulation, 54:*826, 1976.

148. Dietary Fat and Coronary Disease: Leading Article. *Br Med J, ii:*89, 1957.

149. Jepson, E. M.: Hypercholesterolemic xanthomatosis. Treatment with a corn oil diet. *Br Med J, i:*847, 1961.

150. Christakis, G. et al.: The anti-coronary club. A dietary approach to the prevention of coronary heart disease. A seven year report. *Am J Public Health, 56:*299, 1966.

151. Jons, R. J., Klimt, Ch. R., and Stamler, J.: The coronary drug project —

A secondary prevention trial. In Schettler, G. and Weizel, A. (Eds.): *Atherosclerosis III.* Berlin, Springer-Verlag, 1974, p. 729.

152. Clofibrate in ischaemic heart disease. *Br Med J, ii:*765, 1971.
153. Krasno, L. R. and Kidera, G. J.: Clofibrate in coronary heart disease. *JAMA, 219:*845, 1972.
154. Symposium on Atromid. *J Atheroscler Res, 3:* 1963.
155. Buchwald, H.: Ileal bypass in the treatment of the hyperlipidemias. *J Atheroscler Res, 10:*1, 1969.
156. Doll, R. and Peto, R.: Mortality in relation to smoking: 20 years observation on male British doctors. *Br Med J, ii:*1525, 1976.
157. Aronow, W. S.: Smoking, carbon monoxide and coronary heart disease. *Circulation, XLVIII:*1169, 1973.
158. Wald, N., Howard, S., Smith, P. G., and Kjeldsen, K.: Association between atherosclerotic diseases and carboxyhaemoglobin levels in tobacco smokers. *Br Med J, i:*761, 1973.
159. Thomson, J. G.: Production of severe atheroma in a transplanted human heart. *Lancet, ii:*1088, 1969.

CHAPTER 5

THE PREVENTIVE PROGRAMME

THE most persuasive evidence for the institution of programmes for the prevention of coronary heart disease come from studies of the incidence in native born and migrant populations. This has been conclusively demonstrated with native South Koreans and those that have migrated to the United States and in the Bantu populations in South Africa.

At least three risk factors are now firmly established; they are blood pressure, serum cholesterol levels, and cigarette smoking. The problem with the first two is to define normal acceptable limits, and it seems most likely that the acceptable norm for plasma cholesterol is too high. Any proposed preventative programme, of necessity, would have to be applied widely without rigid definition of persons at risk. For example, to identify the population at risk in the United States would cost billions of dollars in terms of laboratory and other investigations.

There is little doubt that success of primary prevention will be best achieved if it is started early in childhood. For example, in the Netherlands, where the incidence of ischaemic heart disease is alarmingly high, 10 to 30 percent of preschool children have been shown to be hyperlipidemic. Not many centres have tackled atherosclerosis as a paediatric problem, but there are trials in Louisiana and Arizona (1).

Of the three main risk factors, the lowering of cholesterol levels seems most feasible. Even this meets with the opposition of food faddists who encourage the consumption of milk, eggs, and meat to promote health. For this and other reasons, the preventive project needs to be international, involving a radical change of dietary habits that are ingrained in various races.

Perhaps the easiest thing to do is to reduce the total amount of fat in the diet so that the amount of calories contributed by fat is lowered from 40 to 30 percent. In particular, the reduction should be aimed at saturated fats such as butter and fat meat as well as hydrogenated oils of either fish or vegetable origin. If the individual is obese, a reduction of total calorie intake is desirable; this includes not only fat but also alcohol and cane sugar, which are rich sources of calories.

The problem of lowering fat intake is that most of Western cookery involves fat. If these fats are reduced it might be well to replace them with polyunsaturated fats to secure the compliance of the subject. The precise details of the diets that have been used are described in many of the books, pamphlets, and reports that have been issued over the past years (2).

If, despite diet, the plasma cholesterol levels remain in the range of 275 to 300 mgm/dl, thought should be given to adding a hypocholesterolemic drug to the regime. This should not be done until the physician is satisfied that there has been strict compliance by the patient with the dietary instructions. It is often wise to seek the aid of a dietician before instituting drug therapy.

Hypertriglyceridemia usually indicates an excessive intake of calories either in the form of carbohydrate or alcohol; if so, dietary measures are required. The intake of these dietary ingredients should be drastically reduced. If there is an associated hypercholesterolemia, the same regime is applied as for hypercholesterolemia alone.

Half of the deaths of smokers are due to cardiovascular disease, which is not surprising because many people still smoke and cardiovascular disease is common. However, there is a well-defined association between cigarette smoking and myocardial infarction and an even closer one with peripheral vascular disease and intermittent claudication. Pipe and cigar smokers are less vulnerable to arterial disease, but unfortunately, it is not true that a change from cigarettes to pipes and cigars is beneficial. This is probably because the erstwhile cigarette smoker continues to inhale. Nevertheless, as a last resort, if the smoker cannot be dissuaded, a change to a pipe might reap some slight benefit. Other alternatives include advice not to smoke more than five cigarettes a day and to use filter cigarettes or the new smoking mixtures, which have a low content of nicotine.

No drug has yet been found that successfully prevents smoking. Simple firm advice by the doctor to his patient is the

only way of dealing with the problem. Patients who have suffered a myocardial infarction will show a 60 percent compliance with instructions to stop smoking. This usually lasts
for at least one year.

The important role of elevated blood pressure as an atherogenic agent has already been identified, and it appears that the
systolic pressure is as useful a predicator as the diastolic.

About 40 percent of middle-aged men have diastolic pressures
of 90 mm Hg or more, and this situation needs remedy. Some
confusion exists about levels of blood pressure because of the
end point of the auscultatory sounds used to record it. Some use
muffling, others disappearance of Korotkoffs's sounds. The
latter gives a diastolic pressure about 5 mm lower than the
former. In addition, blood pressure varies during the day, is
higher in hospital than at home, and tends to fall with frequent
visits by the physician. Nevertheless, the medical profession
takes too lax a view of the serious role of hypertension in
ischaemic heart disease, and the treatment of hypertension is
often delayed until symptoms appear. Furthermore, dosage of
hypotensive drugs is not properly controlled, and blood pressure measurements are erratic and often not done under optimal conditions. It is no wonder that studies of the effects of
control of hypertension on ischaemic heart disease are confused
and inconclusive.

It is important to keep in mind that for every 10 mm Hg
above "normal" the risk of ischaemic heart disease in men in
their forties rises by 20 percent. This risk is multiplied by
smoking, hypercholesterolemia, and inactivity. The presence of
left ventricular hypertrophy also has an adverse effect.

Many doctors dislike using hypotensives, particularly in persons with symptomless hypertension, because of the alleged
side effects. The patient must be warned to accept side effects
initially if effective blood pressure control is to be achieved. For
example, a-methyldopa, which is an effective hypotensive particularly in conjunction with small doses of a diuretic, will
initially produce faintness, dryness of the mouth, and so on.
When the patient has adjusted his life-style, for example, by not
jumping to his feet from a sitting position but by rising slowly,
much of the giddiness and faintness goes away. Side effects

such as haemolytic anaemia, liver damage, etc. are rare and inconsequential in comparison with the effectiveness of the drug.

The main benefits of hypotensive agents are in the prevention of stroke and left ventricular failure. This is not surprising because the strain has been taken off the cardiovascular tube. The United States Veterans Administration Trials showed no beneficial effect of treatment on the incidence of myocardial infarction (3). These men were treated late. The effects of early treatment of hypertension will undoubtedly show a different influence on the incidence of ischaemic heart disease.

The effects of trying to deal with obesity, physical inactivity, and environmental stress are not clear. When these factors are related to hypertension, as they often are, the management of both conditions is of value. The same applies to diabetic patients who often are obese, hypertensive, and hyperlipidemic. There is, at present, no evidence that proper control of diabetes has any effect upon the incidence of coronary heart disease in these subjects. However, the treatment of the associated risk factors is of value.

There is little evidence to support the value of dietary fibre in the control of ischaemic heart disease. Nor is there any evidence that cane sugar has an adverse effect save by promoting obesity. Coffee seems to be harmless from this point of view and so does alcohol. However, the latter is a potent source of calories and leads readily to hypertriglyceridemia, though this, of itself, is not related to the pathogenesis of coronary heart disease. There is, regrettably, no convincing evidence that alcohol exerts any independent protective effect.

The role of dietary salt is controversial. It is a good rule to avoid excess and particularly not to add it to infant foods. There is little doubt that the high incidence of cerebral haemorrhage among the Japanese was associated with the high level of dietary salt. Changing dietary habits, in Japan, are leading to a fall in the incidence of stroke. There is much experimental evidence to support the hypertensive role of dietary salt. One of the most effective ways of producing hypertension, in the rat, is to remove about one third of the total kidney tissue and then to feed a high-salt diet. Dietary salt should be treated as one would a drug — the dosage must be closely watched. There is no reason to doubt that a nationwide reduction of intake would reduce the incidence of coronary heart disease.

Soft drinking water has been associated with an increased incidence of ischaemic heart disease. How soft, acid water exerts its effect is unknown. It may be that it dissolves lead, cadmium, and chromium easier than does hard water. In this respect, cadmium has been associated with hypertension, and it may be the *modus operandi* of soft water. So far as prevention of heart disease is concerned, it is negligible. The less said further to unnerve the bewildered patient the better.

Children present a special problem in the prevention of heart disease. All the risk factors are found and Type II hyperlipoproteinaemia, for example, can be detected in the first year of life. Hypertension is rare in children, partly because the blood pressure is not measured. It is important to keep an eye on those whose parents are hypertensive or have suffered some hypertensive complication. Physicians should look afresh at the evidence linking ischaemic heart disease and hypertension and pursue a more vigorous attack upon it even in childhood, should it be indicated. The foundations of atherosclerosis are laid in childhood, and indecisive dithering by the doctor can lead to irreparable arterial injury. In general, children should not be regarded independently of their parents, for their risk factors are often shared by the rest of the family (4).

Having discussed a possible prevention programme, the question arises as to how it should be initiated. First of all, much can be done by the use of mass media for advertisement of healthier ways of living. This must be done carefully. People, especially the young, ignore the dire warning of their elders and doctors. A subtle approach is required to persuade a nation to change its eating and drinking habits, to exercise properly, and to accept treatment even when no symptoms exist.

Secondly, the key figure in the promulgation of the programme is the general practitioner. He knows the family, recognises their genetic and environment hazards, and can gently ease them towards reduction of risk and acceptance of drug treatment should it be necessary. Unfortunately, family doctors are getting fewer. Most general practitioners are heavily involved in the treatment of the sick and particularly of the elderly. The time available to them for health education of their families is often severely curtailed by pressure of therapeutic work. Departments of Health Education are, at present, in their infancy. They need strengthening by the professional expertise of doctors if they are to propagate a persuasive effective role in the community.

A number of trials have been launched in various countries in Europe under the auspices of the World Health Organization (5). The project started in 1970 and consisted of a study of the methods involved in launching multifactorial preventive trials. By 1976 the trials were going ahead, but the collection of the end point results of coronary heart disease was not complete. An important aspect of the work was the standardisation of the laboratory methods for measuring various parameters such as cholesterol and other lipids. This was done at the W.H.O. lipid reference centre in Prague. In addition, an Electrocardiogram Coding Centre has been set up in Budapest to standardise results for computer analysis.

Studies at the different centres in Europe varied from place to place, being designed to meet the local conditions. One or two general points have emerged so far. The effects of screening the population itself are controversial. Experience from the Zagreb study suggests that screening alone may cause a reduction in the level of risk factors in the community, but data from Gothenburg did not support this view. The United Kingdom project emphasised the importance of the challenge of personal contact to achieve changes in behaviour. In general, the greatest success was, as might be expected, in those persons who are at high risk and who had received intensive counselling, as in the Oslo study.

The programme in Zurich was designed to test the effects of intensive health education using mass media. Another group of people not subjected to propaganda was used as a control. The results of this trial are being evaluated. Considerable success has been achieved in Eastern Finland where the incidence of myocardial infarction was 14 percent per 1000 among males aged thirty to sixty-four. Using intensive methods of general and personal propaganda, they have succeeded in decreasing current smokers by 12 percent, in promoting the use of low-fat milk in 48 percent of the population, and in persuading 50 percent of males to have regular measurements of blood pressure. During the trial, the percentage on antihypertensive therapy increased from 3.1 to 9.1 percent.

Results from Gothenburg, in Sweden, have also been satisfactory in general. Postal questionnaires were sent out, and those who refused to participate were characterised by a high incidence of alcoholic problems and a higher mortality from ischaemic heart disease. It was surprising how unaware the Swedish population was of the relationship of coronary artery disease and smoking, despite widespread publicity of the facts. It may well be that the intensive campaign that purported to show no relation between smoking and ischaemic heart disease in twin studies may have influenced the general attitude. The trial in the United Kingdom consisted of advice in diet and smoking, weight reduction, and the encouragement of physical activity. Hypotensive drugs were used if the mean of four systolic pressure readings was more than 160 mm Hg. It will be interesting to see the results, which have yet to be published. The level of blood pressure chosen is far too high, and it might be expected that the results of the trial will be equivocal. At least it may serve to indicate the importance of hypertension as a prime cause of ischaemic heart disease. The Italian trial, in Rome, had a more positive attack on hypertension. Not only were hypotensives used, but a low-caloric, low-salt diet was instituted as well for those with hypertension. They also used drugs to control hypertriglyceridemia and hyperuricemia.

The Belgian project was concerned to identify major risk factors as well as a psychosocial questionnaire. In Poland, the high-risk subjects were variously referred to special clinics such as Metabolic Disturbance, Anti-hypertensive, and Anti-smoking clinics. As in other trials, the best results were achieved in the high-risk subjects, but overall the results were poor. It proved especially difficult to achieve reduction of weight and cholesterol levels.

Oslo studies accepted a lower level of systolic pressure (150 mm Hg) for the institution of hypotensive therapy, which was initially hydrochlorthiazide followed by α-methyldopa if a satisfactory drop of blood pressure was not achieved. In all the trials reported to date, the main prongs of the prevention programme are the control of hypertension and serum cholesterol and the abolition of smoking and, for the future, it is unlikely that many significant factors will be added. It is best to concentrate on a few rather than on many factors. There is a limit to human compliance.

References

1. Reynolds, J. L.: Modification of atherosclerotic disease risk factors in children. *J Louisiana Med Soc, 124:*353, 1972.
2. Prevention of coronary heart disease. Report of a joint working party. *J R Coll Physicians, Lond, 10:* 1976.
3. Veterans administration cooperative study group. Effects of treatment on morbidity in hypertension. *JAMA, 213:*1152, 1970.
4. Lloyd, J. K. and Wolff, O. H.: A paediatric approach to the prevention of atherosclerosis. *J Atheroscler Res, 10:*135, 1969.
5. The Prevention of Coronary Disease. Report of a working group. Regional Office for Europe, W.H.O., Copenhagen, 1977.

CHAPTER 6

MEASUREMENT OF ATHEROSCLEROSIS

A FUNDAMENTAL component of the animal experimental and human studies that we have discussed in this book is the accurate mensuration of degrees of atheroma in vessels *in vivo* and at postmortem examination. The most difficult problem is measurement in the living animal and in particular in man. It might be thought that the delineation and measurement of areas of atherosclerosis in an opened, fixed aorta might be easy, yet it is surprising how variable are the results when different methods are used.

In 1964, Granston et al. (1) compared planimetric and visual assessment of degrees of atherosclerosis in the aortas of 452 persons obtained at postmortem. They recognised four types of lesion after sudan staining: (a) flat sudanophilic, (b) raised sudanophilic, (c) raised nonsudanophilic (fibrous plaque), (d) complicated showing ulceration, thrombosis, haemorrhage, or calcification.

Granston et al. outlined the lesions using tracing paper and measured their area by a rolling wheel planimeter, making two readings of each area and then dividing by two. They compared this with the visual method and showed a large error in visual assessment alone. Furthermore, they showed that visual results varied on successive observations of the same specimen and also when the same observer made repeated estimations.

On the other hand, Solberg et al. (2) used unaided visual estimation of the extent of atherosclerosis in cerebral arteries. This was part of a large international study. They emphasised that careful control of the conditions under which the arteries were prepared is imperative, and furthermore, experience and training were essential if the observers were to obtain reproducible results.

Another method of measuring the extent and distribution of lesions in relation to emerging ostia of vessels is to stain and photograph aortic lesions. The photographs are then projected onto polar coordinates the orifice being centred on the polar grid. Zero degrees was the upstream coordinate and 180° downstream. When the results were plotted as rectangular coordinates, the area and distribution of lesions could be readily determined (3).

Other morphometric methods involve the use of graticules applied to the vessel surface and counting the number of squares overlying areas of atheroma (4). Another refinement is to photograph the lesions in the aorta that have been stained by sudan dyes. A sheet of clear cellulose acetate paper, in which holes have been punched at regular intervals, is then placed over the photograph. This is the method of point counting that has wide applications for the measurement of many biological variables. The principle is that a large number of points are scattered over irregular outlines on a plane surface and that the number of points over these outlines is proportional to their area. Clearly the principle error of the method depends upon the total number of points counted (5).

Most of the methods that we have described provide reliable ways of measuring the extent of atherosclerotic disease, particularly in the experimental animal. It is not so easy in the human subject where the aorta may be calcified and consequently cannot readily be flattened for accurate measurements to be made. Measurements of area provide no evidence of the degree of occlusion. This is the more important aspect of disease, particularly in the coronary arteries. Techniques for measuring degrees of occlusion are varied. Some of the early studies were made by Schlesinger by injecting radiopaque material into the coronary arteries (6). Only in recent times have techniques been developed that enable casts to be made of coronary arteries and the vessels still preserved for macroscopic examination of their inner surfaces (7). Basically, a semirigid polyester cast is used with less than 3 percent shrinkage. Copper is incorporated into the resin, which makes it radiopaque. A parting agent is also added to allow easy separation of the cast from the vessel without causing damage. The study of angiograms, the casts, and the vessel wall itself enabled an accurate assessment of the degree of coronary occlusion.

Crawford et al. (8), in a series of papers, have refined the angiographic method. Casts were made of the coronary arteries of human excised hearts by filling them with radiopaque silicone rubber that polymerises rapidly. Segments were marked off on the angiograms, and the corresponding intimal surface of the artery was graded visually. Using a film digitizer computer, they located the vessel edges on the angiograms and estimated the degree of atherosclerosis from deviations in the smoothness of the edge. There was a close correlation of this method with the visual grading of atheroma.

This method holds a good deal of promise for the angiographic assessment of arterial disease in man. It works well with leg arteries and detects early lesions, which are the ones most likely to regress and are, therefore, of considerable interest to this discussion. At present it is more difficult to apply the method to coronary arteries because of their perpetual motion and also because of their complex shape and configuration.

The same authors have used the computer controlled image dissector to study changes in the femoral arteries of patients with treated hyperlipoproteinaemia. They were able to detect regression of lesions in nine, progression in thirteen and no change in three after a period of thirteen months. In the patients whose angiograms had improved, there were significant falls in blood cholesterol, triglycerides, and in blood pressure. No such changes occurred in those whose lesions had progressed (9).

The application of fibre optic and reflection spectrophotometry has enabled studies to be made of the degree of aortic atheroma *in vivo*. The principle depends on colour differences between atheromatous plaques and the normal aortic wall, which yield different reflection spectra. A fibre probe is inserted into the aorta consisting of two fibre bundles. One provides illumination of the inner aortic wall, and the other transmits the reflected light to a measuring device outside the body. On the whole, the method is satisfactory. There are occasional design difficulties in the probes, which preclude good optical contact between the probe and the aortic wall; in jaundiced patients the method is, of course, inapplicable (10).

There has been no lack of ingenuity in the many and varied attempts to measure atheroma. Chemical estimates of lipids or calcium have been used by some. More recently, chemical methods have been applied to measure the extent of atheroma *in vivo*. One such method is the intravenous injection of ^{123}I labelled fibrinogen followed by examination of the neck region with the gamma camera. This showed uptake of fibrinogen by atherosclerotic plaques. This is a temporary event and disappears within twenty hours of the injection. It is also likely that fibrinogen is only taken up by older plaques so that the method may not be helpful in detecting earlier lesions. Studies with radioactive platelets might produce better results (11). Others have used callipers that measure the thickness of vessel walls at various points.

Unfortunately, Gertsen's statement is still true: "Although research on atherosclerosis has reached tremendous dimensions during the last fifty years, the basic problem of grading atherosclerosis has not yet been solved" (12).

References

1. Cranston, W. I., Mitchell, J. R. A., Russell, R. W. R., and Swartz, C. J.: The assessment of aortic disease. *J Atheroscler Res, 4:*29, 1964.
2. Solberg, L. A., Moosy, J., Williams, O. D., Guzman, M. A., and McGarry, P. A.: Evaluation of atherosclerotic lesions in cerebral arteries by unaided visual estimation. *Atherosclerosis, 16:*155, 1972.
3. Cornhill, J. F. and Roach, M. R.: Quantitative method for the evaluation of atherosclerotic lesions. *Atherosclerosis, 20:*131, 1974.
4. Al-Hishimi, A. S. and Williams, G.: A morphometric method for assessment of atherosclerotic lesions. *Atherosclerosis, 14:*401, 1971.
5. Mitchell, J. R. A. and Cranston, W. I.: A simple method for the quantitative assessment of aortic disease. *J Atheroscler Res, 5:*135, 1965.
6. Schlesinger, M. J.: New radiopaque mass for vascular injection. *Lab Invest, 6:*1, 1957.
7. Robbins, S. L. and Fish, S. J.: A new angiographic technique providing a simultaneous permanent cast of the coronary lumen. *Am J Clin Pathol, 42:*156, 1964.
8. Crawford, D. W., Beckenbach, E. S., Blankenhorn, D. H., Selzer, R. H., and Brooks, S. H.: Grading of coronary atherosclerosis. Comparison of a modified IAP visual grading method and a new quantitative angiographic technique. *Atherosclerosis, 19:*231, 1974.
9. Barndt, R., Blankenhorn, D. H., Crawford, D. W., and Brooks, S. H.: Regression and progression of early femoral atherosclerosis in treated hyperlipoproteinemic patients. *Ann Intern Med, 86:*139, 1977.
10. Edholm, P. and Jacobson, B.: Detection of aortic atheromatosis in vivo by

reflection spectrophotometry. *J Atheroscler Res,* 5:592, 1965.
11. Mettinger, K. L., Larsson, S., Ericson, K., and Casseborn, S.: Detection of atherosclerotic plaques in carotid arteries by the use of ^{123}I-fibrinogen. *Lancet, i*:242, 1978.
12. Gertsen, J. C.: Atherosclerosis in an autopsy series. *Acta Pathol Microbiol Scand Suppl, 170:*1, 1974.

POSTCRIPT

THIS is the first book on the subject of regressing atherosclerosis; many more will undoubtedly follow as knowledge unfolds. A great deal has been learned about atheroma in the past fifty years, but much of it needs revision, repetition, and refinement.

For example, Stender et al.[1] have reconsidered their view that carbon monoxide increases the uptake of cholesterol by the arterial wall. Adams[2] has clarified the problem of regression of atherosclerosis in the rabbit and concludes that mild degrees of the disease can regress in this experimental animal. Polyunsaturated fats will reverse cholesterol-adrenaline-induced atheroma in the rhesus monkey[3].

The basic principles stand firm. What is needed is more detailed knowledge of the pathophysiology of the progression of atherosclerosis from its earliest beginnings. Given this, an attack on prevention and regression can be mounted with more scientific certainty than at present.

---

[1]Stender, S., Astrup, P., and Kjeldsen, K.: The effect of carbon monoxide on cholesterol in the aortic wall. *Atherosclerosis, 28:*357, 1977.

[2]Adams, C. W. M. and Morgan, R. S.: Regression of atheroma in the rabbit. *Atherosclerosis, 28:*399, 1977.

[3]Chakravarti, R. N., Sasi-Kumar, B., Nair, C. R., and Kumar, M.: Reversibility of cholesterol-adrenaline induced atherosclerosis in rhesus monkeys. Evaluation of safflower oil and low-fat low-calorie diet. *Atherosclerosis, 28:*405, 1977.

NAME INDEX

A

Abdulla, Y. H., 58, 76
Acosta, D., 77
Adams, C. W. M., 12-13, 24-25, 39, 58, 70, 76, 93
Agmon, J., 34
Ahmed, S. S., 73
Al-Hishimi, A. S., 91
Albrecht, 39
Alexander, A. F., 73
Alexander, K. M., 27
Alfin-Slater, R. B., 71
Allalouf, D., 34
Almy, T. P., 74
Alper, R., 26
Altschul, R., 50, 72, 74
Amplatz, K., 8
Anderson, J. T., 34
Angell, C., 24
Anitschkow, N., 16, 38, 70
Antonius, J. I., 26
Aono, S., 76
Aravanis, C., 34
Armitage, A. K., 73
Armstrong, M. L., 40, 71
Aronow, W. S., 79
Aschoff, L., 3, 7
Astrup, P., 48, 70, 73-74, 93 fnt.
Augustyn, J. M., 71

B

Bailey, J. M., 77
Bar, A., 76
Barker, N. W., 7
Barlow, G. H., 27
Barndt, R., 5, 8, 91
Bayliss, O. B., 24-25, 70
Beckenbach, E. S., 91
Beitzke, H., 3, 7
Bell, F. P., 24, 26

Bellon, E. R., 74
Bender, S. R., 75
Benditt, E. P., 25
Benditt, J. M., 25
Bensley, S. H., 25
Benyo, R., 71
Berenson, G. S., 25
Berger, F. M., 56, 76-77
Berkson, D. M., 35
Bernick, S., 71
Besterman, E. M. M., 77
Bierman, E. L., 78
Bing, R. J., 24, 73
Biozzi, G., 75
Birnbaum, P. S., 78
Biss, K., 35
Blackburn, H., 34
Blackshear, P. J., 77
Blankenhorn, D. H., 8, 91
Blaton, B., 58, 76
Block, Y. E., 77
Boissel, J. P., 78
Boissou, H., 78
Bondjers, G., 18, 26, 70
Bonnett, L., 49, 73
Booth, J., 70
Boother, J., 76
Börkerud, S., 18, 26, 70
Bortz, W. M., 70
Bouisson, 64
Bourdillon, M. C., 78
Bourne, C., 72
Bourne, G. H., 8
Bowyer, D. E., 26, 75
Boyd, G. S., 76
Boyle, A. J., 77
Branwood, A. W., 60, 77
Brass, I. D., 72
Brest, A. N., 75
Bronte-Stewart, B., 34
Brooks, S. H., 8, 91
Brown, B. W., 75

95

Tennent, D. M., 76
Thomas, W. A., 26
Thomsen, H. K., 48, 73
Thomson, J. G., 79
Thorne, M. C., 35
Tillmanns, H., 24, 73
Toki, K., 76
Toor, M., 34
Topping, D. L., 48, 73
Tracy, R. E., 14, 25
Tromp, S. W., 76
Tucker, C. G., 42, 71
Turner, D. M., 48, 73
Turner, D. R., 25
Turney, S. W., 76
Turto, H., 73

U

Uitto, J., 73

V

Vallance-Owen, J., 74, 78
Van Buchem, F. S. P., 34
Van Winkle, M., 54, 70, 75
Vaniitallie, T. B., 76
Varco, R. L., 8, 77
Vasquez, J. M., 24
Vesselinovitch, D., 7, 71, 74, 78
Vihert, A. M., 7

W

Wagner, W. D., 59, 77
Wald, N., 79
Wallace, W. M., 71
Wanstrup, J., 73-74
Warmanen, E. L., 71

Wartman, A., 77
Weber, G., 70
Wegelius, O., 25
Wehrle, C. L., 75
Weizel, A., 20, 25, 75-76, 79
Weiss, H. S., 30, 34
Welsh, J. J., 74
Wenzel, D. G., 77
Werthessen, N. T., 26
Whitney, L. H., 34
Widdowson, 43
Wigand, G., 71
Wilens, S. L., 7, 24
Will, D. H., 73
Williams, G., 91
Williams, J. L., 35
Williams, O. D., 91
Wilson, R. B., 26
Winter, M. O., Jr., 4, 7
Wissler, R. W., 7, 20, 26, 35, 40, 64, 71, 74, 77-78
Withering, William, 45
Wolf, P. A., 35
Wolff, O. H., 87
Wolinsky, H., 23
Wood, P. D. S., 75

Y

Yant, W. P., 73
Younger, R., 76
Youroukova, K., 25
Yudkin, 32, 65

Z

Zhoanov, V. S., 7
Ziegler, D. D., 74
Zollman, P. E., 77

SUBJECT INDEX

arterial endothelium, 15-19
arterial lipids, 10-13
arterial mucopolysaccharides, 13-14
arterial smooth muscle, 19-21
blood coagulation, 21-23
components of, 9-27
role in atherogenesis, 9-27
increased uptake of radioactively labelled carbon, 11
inflammatory component, 14-15
vessel wall, 9-10
Atherosclerotic plaques, 12, 14-15
ATPase activity, 61
Avocado pear, 45

B

Baboons, 21, 44, 55, 57
Balloon catheter, 42
Bantu populations, 80
Beagle hounds, 50
Behaviour patterns, 30-31
Belgian project, 86
Bell Telephone System, 31
Benzyl-N-benzyl carbethoxyhydroxamate, 58
Binding of bile acids in the gut, 56
Birds, 30, 53
Blackgram
carbohydrate fraction, 45
effects of, 44-45
globulin fraction, 44-45
Blood cholesterol, 90
Blood coagulation, 38, 55
atherogenesis and, 21-23
Blood group A, 33
Blood group O, 33
Blood platelets (*see* Platelets)
Blood pressure, 32, 68, 80, 82, 86-87, 90
Bovine serum albumen, injections of, 54-55
Bradykinin, 60
British civil servants, 68
British doctors, 69
Bus conductors, 29
Butter, 80
Butter fat, 65

C

Cadmium, 33, 84

Calcification, 88
Calorie intake, 64-65
excessive, 81
reduction in, 3, 81
Cane sugar, 81, 83
Carbohydrate metabolism, abnormalities of, 52
Carbohydrates, 44, 81
Carbon monoxide inhalation, 47-49, 69, 93
Carboxyhaemoglobin (COHb), 69
level in blood of smokers, 37
Cardiovascular disease, 81
Cardiovascular disease risk, 69
Cardiovascular tissue culture conference, 60
Carotenoid compound, 60
Carotid sinus area of internal carotid artery, 7
Casein, 44
Catabolism, 37
Catecholamines, 10
Cell turnover, 17
Cellular proliferation, 21
Central Europe, decline in incidence of atherosclerosis in, 3
Cerebral hemorrhage, 3
Chelating agents, 59
Chemical estimates of lipids or calcium, 90-91
Chickens, 30-31, 60
Chicks, 38, 51-53, 57
Children, 84
Chlorpheniramine, 59
Cholesterol, 10, 29, 37
accumulation of, 11
disassociation from its lipoprotein vehicle, 12
role of uptake of, 11
Cholesterol absorption, 67
Cholesterol-acetate, implantation of, 12
Cholesterol esters, 11, 37
hydrolysis of, 19
intra-aortic insertion, 12
intraperitoneal insertion, 12
Cholesterol feeding, 38-39
cessation of, 38-39
Cholesterol-induced lesions, 30
Cholestyramine, 40, 51, 56, 60, 67
Chondroitin polysulphate, 61